LIVE WELL

LIVE
WELL

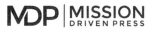

Empowering Habits for Vibrant Health
and Unstoppable Energy

Adriana Shuman

MDP | MISSION
DRIVEN PRESS

Published by Mission Driven Press, an imprint of Forefront Books, Nashville, Tennessee.
Distributed by Simon & Schuster.

Library of Congress Control Number: 2025902143

Print ISBN: 978-1-63763-404-2
E-book ISBN: 978-1-63763-405-9

Cover Design by Bruce Gore, Gore Studio, Inc.
Interior Design by Bill Kersey, KerseyGraphics

Printed in the United States of America

To you, dear reader, my friend—may this book inspire and empower you to create lasting, vibrant health with ease. I hope it helps you truly understand your body and environment, guiding you to take charge of your well-being in a way only you can.

CONTENTS

THE JOURNEY TO HEALTH

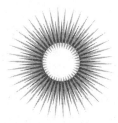

If life is a journey, each attempt to step forward depends on how well—or how poorly—you take care of yourself. The choices you make can either propel you toward great vitality or eventually drag you into disease. Neglect your health, and you'll feel the weight of fatigue and illness. Embrace a healthier lifestyle, and you'll find boundless energy to achieve your dreams. I've experienced both sides of this story.

I was born into a communist country in Bratislava, Czechoslovakia, which became Slovakia in 1993 after the Velvet Revolution. We lived on the second floor of an eight-story apartment building. On the surface, I had everything I needed to be happy—a prominent scientist father and a mother who cooked delicious meals daily, worked, and kept our home spotless. Beneath what seemed like a great family life, my own life was overshadowed by my father's violence and rage and my mother's abuse, lies, and manipulations, which inflicted deep, severe trauma on me.

Living in constant fear, unsure of what would occur in my home day to day, hour to hour, moment to moment, resulted in numerous health challenges for me. As a child, I would hide in my bedroom with the door closed, bracing my soul for my parents' next outburst, hoping this time my mother would not pull me out of my room to protect her from the yelling and beating.

Growing up during Communism, life was bleak and oppressive. As a child, I developed a variety of health issues. Constantly living in fear and chronic stress, my immune system was compromised. Since infancy, I had often been prescribed antibiotics for one reason or another. I experienced two brain injuries from falls early in life, leading to more trauma and adding to my learning disabilities. It terribly affected the memory center in my brain. I was told I was lucky to survive the first fall. I was sick physically and emotionally.

Looking back, the cause of many of my problems was chronic stress and trauma. I realize unhealthy food played a huge role in my poor health as well. My mother was an amazing cook, but our meals consisted of a lot of fried food and were high in processed carbohydrates—a lot of bread, fried cheese, white rice, and weekly freshly baked goods my mom loved to make. Fresh, plant-fiber-rich foods were rarely on the dining table. There was always plenty of sugar in the house too. My dad would often buy not one bar, but an entire box of twelve milk chocolate bars for me, which I'd eat within a week or two. We had delicious, rich soups and crepes with jam and chocolate syrup for lunch. That's simply the way it was, and we didn't know anything about nutrition, gut health, or proper hydration.

The lack of proper nutrition wasn't the entire problem. My parents compelled me to eat much more than I needed, even when I cried out that I was full. My father had been traumatized growing up during World War II, never having enough food after the early death of his parents. He was poor and all alone, left to fend for himself in a war-torn country. My mother experienced a similar fate. So, for them, it was important to always eat more, and to always make sure I had enough in my belly, just in case. For my parents, it was essentially a sin to throw away food.

Years later, during my final year of pharmacy school, I took the first steps on my journey to health. As I learned more about the pharmaceutical industry and stood behind the pharmacy counter for the first time, I had an uncomfortable feeling—a deep, undeniable feeling in my soul: I wasn't meant to be in this industry. The idea of dispensing medication after medication sickened me. I wanted to help people heal naturally and more effectively. There is a time and place for pharmaceutical prescription drugs, but I knew deep inside that health is not created in the pharmaceutical lab but rather at home with our lifestyle and beliefs.

At that time, however, that feeling in my soul was a quiet, distant voice. I had a different priority: to escape the terror that had completely enveloped my first twenty-six years of life. With the help of my closest friends, I fled to the United States, arriving in New York in 2001 with little English, a few thousand dollars, and a heart full of pain and hope.

My own health challenges and the loss of many family members to cancer awakened me even more to the importance of a holistic approach to health. I realized that true health is a lifestyle and mindset applied every day, not just when we're sick. I recognized the dangers of America's industrial food complex and wanted to help people escape this vicious cycle. I had lost my grandmother too soon to cancer. Within a few years, I also lost my aunt, my uncle, my father, and, more recently, my best friend. Their bodies had surely been damaged by the unwavering climate of fear, beliefs, and chronic stress in our country, but dangerous habits and poor food choices undoubtedly destroyed their health. Most of them smoked, drank alcohol, and ate fried, sugary, and refined, carbohydrate-rich foods. Their early deaths weren't the result of one factor—they all perished before their time due to lack of a whole-body holistic connection.

If I was going to help people to become healthy, I needed to heal myself first. Through lifestyle tweaks, mindset shifts, and constant curiosity, I eventually felt better than ever before. Since then, I've helped many amazing people heal themselves, and it's been an honor.

My lifelong quest is to understand the human body and create optimal health for myself, my loved ones, and my clients. Results don't come from magic potions, fad diets, or trendy nutrition plans. True health comes from understanding the fundamental principles of our body, mind, and spirit.

I wrote this book to spread my message of health further because I want everyone to live well. My purpose is simple: I want you to learn the truth about achieving strong and long-lasting health; shedding old, unhealthy habits; and living well—not for a few months or years, but for the rest of your beautiful, precious life.

To live well is to live a fulfilling and satisfying life characterized by strength, happiness, and overall well-being on your own terms. To live well encompasses physical, emotional, and mental wellness. This means practicing healthy lifestyle habits, building positive relationships, and prioritizing personal growth and self-care.

How do you do all that? It takes desire, commitment, and consistency. The first fundamental step in living well is shifting your mindset from disease prevention to health creation. Within these pages you'll discover how to do that. And believe me, if I can do it, so can you.

Don't let my background fool you. Yes, I'm a certified functional medicine health coach and a nutritionist with a pharmacy degree from the Faculty of Pharmacy, Comenius University in Bratislava, Slovakia. I've been teaching about healthy, sustainable living since 2008. But I'm not perfect. Far from it. Although I have been able to completely heal from my sugar and processed-carbohydrate addictions, I still enjoy a bar of dark chocolate here and there, and I continue my own healing journey every day. Our purpose as humans isn't to be perfect; it's to live well. I'm confident that if you follow my guidance, you will get there.

Your journey to health and wellness is unique, and it's yours to create. This book is to guide you, to offer the knowledge and tools you need to live well. Embrace the process, be patient with yourself, and know that every step you take is bringing you closer to your dream life. Let's begin this journey together.

Health

Imagine yourself approaching life with zest and purpose. Every morning, you wake up to the soft glow of dawn, greeting the day with gratitude and a nourishing breakfast that fuels your vibrant mitochondria. As you move through your day, you make mindful choices—choosing stairs over elevators, savoring nutrient-rich meals that support your thriving microbiome, and finding moments to meditate and nurture your mental clarity.

Your commitment to a healthy body and mind reflects in your boundless energy and radiant smile as you balance work, play, and meaningful connections. To you, age is just a number, and genetics merely set the stage—your daily choices are the script that shapes your being.

Health isn't a destination but a continuous journey of self-discovery and growth. It's about embracing the harmony between body, mind, and spirit, so you can live fully and impact others positively. You have unwavering belief that every day is an opportunity to thrive.

Health is a word we often hear, but do we truly understand what it means? It's not just about being free from illness or having a fit body. Health goes beyond that. It encompasses our physical, mental, and emotional well-being.

You don't need to be a biologist to understand that living organisms are inside our bodies and real reactions are happening nonstop inside us, affecting how we feel, function, and look. For the most part, we are in control of these processes through our choices—what we eat, think, and do. We are the directors of our health, and our decisions shape the outcomes.

To me, health means having vibrant mitochondria, a thriving microbiome, and a healthy gut lining, which allows me to feel and function great most of my days. It means I can hike with ease, I can travel and carry my luggage, I can get off the ground without using my hands; I have enough energy and strength to do all the things I want to every day of my life.

It's not about age or genetics; by understanding some simple principles, you can feel, function, and look your best until your last day on this beautiful planet. If you want to live well, you have to prioritize and identify what's most important to you.

When we talk about health, the first thing that usually comes to mind is our physical well-being. It's about taking care of our bodies by eating nutritious food, staying active, and getting enough sleep. Physical health is like the foundation of a house—it provides the strength and stability for everything else in our lives.

Health is not just about our bodies. It's also about our minds and emotions. Mental health is equally important. It affects our physical health on every level. It's about having a healthy mindset, being able to cope with stress, and having a sense of purpose and fulfillment in life. Our mental and

Grow your health from the roots up with: The Live Well Method

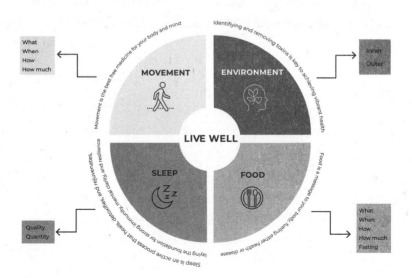

emotional well-being directly impact our overall health and happiness.

Being healthy means finding a balance in all areas of our lives. It's about taking care of our relationships, connecting with others, and having a support system. It's about finding time for activities that bring us joy and relaxation. It's about managing our time and priorities effectively, so we don't feel overwhelmed and stressed all the time.

Health is about more than just surviving; it's about thriving. It's having the energy to chase your dreams, the mental clarity to make wise decisions and the emotional resilience to handle life's challenges with grace. It's about creating a life so rich and fulfilling that every day feels like a gift.

So embrace the journey. Prioritize your health. Make choices that honor your body, mind, and spirit. Because when you truly live well, you not only transform your own life but also inspire those around you to do the same. Remember, true health is the foundation upon which you can build the life you've always dreamed of. Let's embark on this journey together and create the vibrant, fulfilling life you deserve.

MEET THE DREAM TEAM: MITOCHONDRIA AND MICROBIOME (M&M)

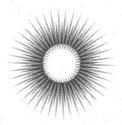

Imagine you have two dear buddies who are dedicated to giving you the very best health and life. One of these friends is an organelle, a crucial part of your cells known as the mitochondria. The other is a thriving community of microorganisms called the microbiome.

Together, this dream team works tirelessly to provide you with energy and make the most of the nutrients you provide them, helping you feel and function at your best every day. When you take care of these two incredible friends, they reward you with an amazing life full of energy and strength. But neglect them, and you invite disease.

The Mitochondria: Your Cellular Powerhouses

Our bodies are made up of cells. Each of your cells, except the red blood cells, contains hundreds or even thousands of these tiny structures, depending on the energy demands of the organ. For example, your heart and brain cells are packed with thousands of mitochondria, given their high energy requirements.

Mitochondria are the power generators of your cells. They are responsible for converting the chemical energy from food (metabolizing food) into a form energy that the cell can use, known as adenosine triphosphate (ATP). Just like a car engine needs fuel to move, mitochondria need fuel to create energy for the body to function. The quality of the material you provide to the mitochondria determines the quality of your daily life. Without mitochondria, there's no power, no life.

Simplified, mitochondria take amino acids from the proteins you eat, fatty acids from the fats you eat, and glucose (a type of sugar) from the carbohydrates you eat, along with the oxygen you breathe, and transform them into the main form of cellular energy, ATP. This complex process requires various vitamins and minerals from your daily food. These *micronutrients* are also known as *coenzymes*—think of them as copilots in this energy production journey. These vital coenzymes are often missing in ultraprocessed factory foods or are added in synthetic forms that your body can't recognize, and therefore can't use.

Energy production in your mitochondria happens constantly, every second of every day. When this process stops, so do you. When it slows down or becomes impaired, so do you. It's quite simple. You feel the effects in your body through unwanted symptoms like headaches, fatigue, lack of focus, memory loss, extra fat, and so much more.

Mitochondria are the powerhouse of every cell, fueling essential functions throughout the body—including the heart. Efficient energy production is critical for maintaining strong, healthy heart muscles. When mitochondria don't function optimally, energy supply to the heart is compromised, leading to conditions like high blood pressure and cardiovascular dysfunction. Beyond energy, mitochondria also regulate lipid metabolism, playing a key role in both cholesterol synthesis and breakdown.

Whether it's the beating of our hearts, the movement of our muscles, or the activity of our brains, it's all possible because our mitochondria are producing energy.

So how does this energy creation actually work? The food you consume is broken down into smaller molecules during digestion. These molecules travel through your bloodstream, entering cells through their lipid membranes. Inside the cells, hundreds or thousands of mitochondria further break down these molecules to generate energy (ATP). This energy is what allows you to read these pages, move around, and live your life.

Remember, the more mitochondria you have and the more efficiently your mitochondria produce energy, the better you feel, function, and look. Take care of them, and they'll take care of you.

The Microbiome: Your Inner Ecosystem

Your body is home to a community of microorganisms—trillions of helpers—that play various roles in supporting your health. This community includes bacteria, fungi, viruses, and other microscopic organisms, collectively known as the microbiome. We rely on them!

Your microbiome covers your skin, inhabits your mouth, and thrives in your large intestine, where the largest number of these incredible little friends work tirelessly. They love you and take care of you if you take care of them.

These microorganisms support your immunity, energy, brain, skin health, sleep, detoxification, weight management, and even the production of hormone neurotransmitters that regulate your mood and emotions. They are at work for the entire system that makes up *you*!

Think of the microbiome like this: What happens when you stop breathing? Your brain and heart eventually stop, and your whole system shuts down. For gut bacteria, their "oxygen" is fiber and polyphenols (found in plants). If you don't give them their "oxygen," they'll die. They are living organisms that need to be fed, and without them, your health suffers.

Microbes facilitate the breakdown of waste we cannot digest, helping eliminate it from the body. The microbiome also breaks down other materials like fibers and complex carbohydrates into simpler molecules like short-chain fatty acids (SCFAs), which are important for creating energy, regulating immune function, and reducing inflammation.

If your gut microbiome is not well-balanced—due to eating ultraprocessed factory foods lacking fiber and polyphenols, chronic stress, a sedentary lifestyle, or an excessive use of antibiotics—its ability to support your immune system and energy levels will be compromised.

Maintaining a healthy microbiome involves removing harmful toxins and having a daily intake of nourishing foods rich in diverse fibers and polyphenols, and eating fermented foods.

We all have a unique composition of the microbiome based on our DNA and our early life experiences, beginning at birth. Research from Cornell University has found that human genetics can significantly influence the functions of the gut microbiome.[1] A mother's microbiome influences newborns through childbirth and breastfeeding, affecting the child's immune system development and susceptibility to diseases in adulthood.

Imbalances in the gut microbiome, such as dysbiosis (an imbalance of beneficial and harmful bacteria), can lead to inflammation and affect every part of the body's function, affecting mitochondria function as well. Moreover, gut health influences nutrient absorption. When the gut lining is compromised (leaky gut), it can lead to systemic inflammation and immune responses that further disrupt hormone balance.

The health of our microbiome is closely linked to heart health. A healthy microbiome can help maintain balanced cholesterol levels, while a disrupted microbiome can contribute to dyslipidemia, an imbalance of lipids (fats) in the blood. Many people don't realize that gut health can significantly impact hormonal balance, which is important for mood regulation, cancer protection, and fertility.

Consider this: You have a union of microorganisms all invested in helping you stay alive and function at your best. These little guys play a crucial role in maintaining various bodily functions such as digestion, hormone production, immune system regulation, fertility, and protection against harmful pathogens.

So how can you help them out?

By nourishing them with the right foods and an optimal lifestyle, you ensure they can keep you in peak condition. This book will help make things simple for you so you can understand how to do this.

How Your Body's Powerhouses and Protectors Work Together for Optimal Wellness

A balanced and diverse microbiome contributes to optimal mitochondrial function by aiding in nutrient absorption and reducing inflammation, both of which are crucial for efficient energy production in mitochondria. Conversely, healthy mitochondria support the maintenance of a resilient and well-functioning microbiome by providing the energy needed for gut cells to function properly, ensuring a healthy environment for beneficial bacteria to thrive. This teamwork enhances overall health and well-being. Therefore, to be healthy, you need to take care of both vital systems.

The mitochondria and microbiome rely on each other, as well as on real food and oxygen, to support our health. When they receive what they need, they work together effectively, allowing you to thrive. Even when life throws unpredictable obstacles your way, a strong and healthy "dream team" of mitochondria and microbiome (M&M) helps you handle these challenges much better. These partners are in constant communication on every level.

Whatever your current health challenges are, begin by investigating the health of your dream team, the M&M. I can't emphasize this enough. Consulting with a trusted healthcare provider—someone who understands the gut-mitochondria connection to overall well-being—is the first step to healing and creating optimal health.

To feel and function at our best, we need to fuel our bodies with high-quality materials. This keeps our mitochondria functioning as powerhouses for our bodies and maintains a thriving microbial community that protects us.

Key Takeaway

When experiencing brain fog, high blood pressure, difficulty losing extra fat, or a lack of energy, think of your dream team inside your body, working hard but becoming exhausted. Consider that your mitochondria and microbiome might be dysfunctional due to an overload of toxins in your body. It's time to change your lifestyle if you want to live well!

All Roads Lead to Mitochondria and Microbiome

As you read these pages, remember that everything connects back to this dream team. Understanding this complex yet simple concept is the key to creating a lifestyle free from harmful beliefs or searching for the miracle pill or newest fad. Instead, you'll live a life filled with robust health and joy.

Healthy microbiome + healthy mitochondria = healthy person. Period.

SIMPLIFIED REPRESENTATION OF THE RELATIONSHIP BETWEEN FOOD, GUT, AND MITOCHONDRIAL FUNCTION

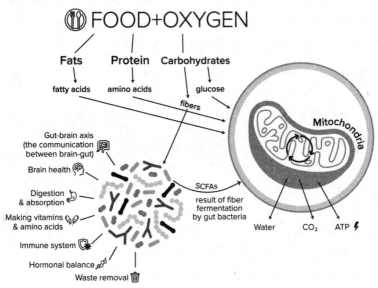

CHAPTER ONE

UNDERSTANDING AND ELIMINATING ENVIRONMENTAL TOXINS

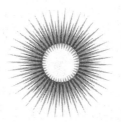

Imagine a charming house in a quaint neighborhood. Outside, it looks like the picture of suburban bliss, with a neatly trimmed lawn and a welcoming front porch. But step inside and it's a different story—complete chaos.

Pipes are leaking, mold creeps up the walls, and the air is thick with dust. Piles of garbage clutter every corner, and mountains of waste block the windows, leaving the rooms in constant darkness.

Despite the chaos, the family living there tries to go about their daily lives. They cook meals in a messy kitchen, dodging heaps of garbage as they search for ingredients. They attempt to relax in a living room buried under layers of trash.

This house is a lot like our bodies when they're overloaded with toxins from the food we eat, stress we feel, and products we use. On the outside, we might look fine, but inside, it's a mess, with dysfunction and inflammation lurking beneath the surface. Toxins interfere with the body's natural processes, weaken the immune system, and leave us feeling tired and sluggish. We carry around extra pounds, deal with headaches, face sleepless nights, and endure other frustrating aches and pains.

Just like the family in the house, we might try to ignore the problem, but it only gets worse with time. The longer we ignore the problem, the more overwhelming it feels. The sooner we acknowledge the need for help, cleansing ourselves of toxins, the sooner we can begin to heal and feel vibrant again.

That's why it's critical for us to discover how to restore our inner sanctuary to its rightful state of harmony and health.

Understanding How Toxins Affect Us

We tend to compartmentalize our bodies and visit different specialists for specific issues: an endocrinologist for thyroid problems, a gut specialist for digestive issues, or a neurologist for memory concerns. Yet we must recognize that organs are interconnected and influence one another.

For example, while an endocrinologist may focus on thyroid function, they might overlook factors like gut microbiome and nutrient absorption, which can impact the thyroid and overall health. Similarly, a gastroenterologist (GI specialist) might address constipation without considering factors like estrogen metabolism or adrenal dysfunction from chronic stress, which could be contributing to the issue.

This segmented approach overlooks the root causes of health issues. The body operates as a complex system where every component—from digestion and hormones to our heart, brain, and thyroid—all work together.

Every system is influenced by what we think, eat, and breathe, and even what we put on our bodies, like lotions and creams. Environmental factors (water, air, soil), personal-care products, and household cleaning supplies influence our well-being. As you can see, what goes into our bodies doesn't only affect the stomach or kidneys, but every cell and system in our bodies.

We are exposed to thousands of toxic substances every day. The average person is exposed to hundreds, if not thousands, of potentially harmful chemicals each day. Like the house filled with trash, if we don't manage these toxins, our bodies can be overrun by garbage. But once we learn what toxins are, how they work, and the real damage they cause, we can remove them from our systems and build a healthier life.

What Is a Toxin?

Let's break it down: Toxins are substances that can cause damage to your cells, including the microbes in your gut. And since your body is made up of cells, every cell can be affected by toxins.

Cells are the basic building blocks of life, responsible for crucial functions like producing energy (ATP), absorbing nutrients, and getting rid of toxins and waste. For example, liver cells are vital for detoxifying harmful substances from your blood. If these cells get damaged, your liver can't function properly, leading to a buildup of toxins in your body.

Oxidation

Toxins cause *oxidation*, which is like rust forming on metal. In your body, oxidation happens when cells interact with oxygen, leading to wear and tear. It's an imbalance between free radicals (unstable molecules that damage cells) and antioxidants (molecules in real, whole foods that neutralize free radicals) in your body.

This wear and tear causes inflammation, which can contribute to diseases like cardiovascular problems, diabetes, cancer, infertility, and more.

Oxidative stress also damages the protective barriers in your blood vessels and gut lining. Think of these barriers as a strong wooden fence protecting a beautiful, peaceful garden. Toxins are like troublemakers trying to dig under the fence and find weak spots to squeeze through, creating openings and causing chaos.

When these barriers are damaged, toxins can pass through and cause damage and inflammation in your tissues and organs. Just as rust weakens metal, oxidation weakens cells, making them less functional.

Toxins can also block receptors on cell membranes, preventing hormones and other important molecules from attaching and triggering responses in your body that are necessary for you to live well. For example, glyphosate, a cancer-causing toxic chemical in the herbicide Roundup, which is used on many crops, can mimic the amino acid glycine. Glycine is crucial for the liver's process of detoxifying the body. If glycine's receptor is blocked by a toxin like glyphosate, it will cause damage to our cells and DNA, which will lead to chronic inflammation and eventually diseases.

Inflammation

Inflammation is like your body's fire alarm system, alerting you to threats. It's a protective response to injury or infection, causing redness, swelling, heat, or pain as your immune system fights off the threat. Acute inflammation is short-term. Whether you get stung by a bee, scrape your knee, or catch a virus, these inflammations are usually not a concern. Of course, we attend to these threats to ensure they don't turn into long-term infections. There are also beneficial forms of inflammation, like when you lift heavy weights at the gym, go for a long run, or use a sauna. These types of short-term inflammation, called hormesis, help our bodies adapt and become stronger.

Chronic inflammation, on the other hand, is long-term and ongoing, and it can be harmful. It can lead to diseases like cancer, infertility, allergies, neurological conditions (like Parkinson's and Alzheimer's), diabetes, mood disorders, and obesity. Daily habits like ingesting alcohol, eating fried foods, or consuming cookies can keep your body in a state of ongoing inflammation.

Chronic inflammation can prevent your organs from functioning properly. For example, an inflamed thyroid can affect your adrenal glands, pancreas, digestion, and liver, leading to aches, extra fat, anxiety, and low mood over time.

If you're constantly dealing with mood issues, headaches, bloating, anxiety, depression, joint pain, acne, irritability, or poor sleep, your body might be inflamed. Symptoms like itchy skin, brain fog, memory loss, asthma, and more are your body's way of letting you know that there is a potential for disease if you do not address the toxic overload that created these issues in the first place.

Symptoms Are Good for You

This is important, so let's repeat it: Symptoms are good for you.

When you hear a creak, see a leak, or notice other noises in your home, you attend to it. It's a sign that something is broken and needs immediate attention. Similarly, symptoms are your body's way of communicating that something is not working well and you should evaluate your lifestyle. Symptoms are messages, acting as a chronic inflammation alarm. When you experience them, it's time to pause and start asking why you're having these symptoms, these alarms, instead of shutting them down with medications.

High blood pressure, diabetes, headaches, infertility, and extra weight are not problems in themselves. They are symptoms of underlying issues—in this case, the toxins in our bodies causing inflammation, resulting in mitochondria and microbiome dysfunction.

Unfortunately, we often convince ourselves that fatigue, headaches, or excess weight are just part of "normal" life, attributing them to genetics or aging. After all, most people have similar problems, so we brush these symptoms off as the price we pay for our modern lifestyles. We think that taking medications will magically make everything "go away." This is what we are being taught.

Disease

Disease is an impaired function caused by chronic inflammation. Disease happens when we keep ignoring these messages, these symptoms. If problems like mold, structural damage, and broken pipes in a house are left unaddressed, eventually the house becomes unlivable.

Remember that diseases like cancer, heart disease, and Alzheimer's take years, even decades, to develop due to poor diet, low activity levels, insufficient sleep, stress, and other negative lifestyle factors that interact with genetics and environment.

Unfortunately, our current healthcare (disease-care) system prioritizes silencing these symptoms with medications because medical professionals often don't know what else to do. The pills don't fix the problem. It's like stepping on a nail and taking a pain pill instead of figuring out the problem, which is the nail, and removing it. The pills numb the pain but don't remove the toxins. We get used to living this way, but that's not okay. We deserve better than this!

That's why we need a different approach to health: addressing the root problems, like removing the nail from the foot. The symptom is not the problem. We should be grateful for the symptoms, since they are our body's way of communicating that something is wrong.

My clients often ask, "Why am I always bloated? Why am I having headaches? Why can't I sleep? What am I doing wrong?" No matter the question, the answer is often the same: It's an overload of toxins. Let's identify where the toxins are coming from, identify the habits that don't serve you well, and create small changes in all areas to eliminate the toxins and propel you to a healthier state.

This is where we will focus on the concept of *prevention*. This simply means developing habits that create health. To focus on prevention, we must shift our mindset from reactive to proactive.

The most critical and urgent thing we can do to help ourselves feel better is to identify and eliminate the toxins that are taking over our bodies. Once we figure out what these toxins are and where they are coming from, we can make choices—not just once, but daily—that will determine the length and quality of our lives.

Toxins (see examples in the Identify Toxins section below) cause **oxidative stress**. **Prolonged oxidative stress** causes cell damage, which then triggers an **inflammatory response**. We feel this inflammation as **symptoms**. If **chronic inflammation** is not addressed with lifestyle changes, it can turn into **disease**.

Where Do Toxins Come From?

Toxins are found in our food and food packaging, water, air, personal care products, electronics, household cleaning products, soil, furniture, and pharmaceutical drugs. Any chemical substances that are foreign to our bodies are called xenobiotics. Our thoughts can be toxic to our bodies too, causing inflammation. Pretty overwhelming, right? And in case that list isn't enough, our bodies also make toxins, also referred to as *endogenous toxins*. These can be substances like urea, which is by breaking down proteins (via ammonia as an intermediate), or homocysteine, which is produced by metabolizing the amino acid methionine. (More on this later.)

Every second, your body's cells are hard at work producing energy so you can go about your daily life. As we learned earlier, this energy is created by tiny organelles within your cells called mitochondria, which convert nutrients from the food you eat into energy.

Heads-up: We're about to get into a slightly more technical explanation about how your body generates energy and handles toxins created during energy production. Don't worry—I'll break it down step-by-step so it's easy to follow. Understanding how these processes work is empowering, and it's a key part of taking control of your own health.

The process of generating energy is a strenuous task for the mitochondria. As mitochondria generate energy, they also produce another endogenous toxin, byproducts known as *reactive oxygen species (ROS)*. These ROS molecules are missing at least one electron, which makes them highly reactive and unstable (free radicals). These free radicals cause damage to cells, including mitochondria themselves, if they are not neutralized.

Thankfully, our bodies have built-in systems, antioxidants like superoxide dismutase (SOD) and glutathione peroxidase (GPx), to help stabilize these free radicals by supplying them with missing electrons.

The problem occurs when there is an imbalance between ROS production and antioxidant levels. That imbalance leads to oxidative stress. This stress, in turn, damages DNA, proteins, and lipids, ultimately contributing to the development of various diseases. How do we support this incredible built-in antioxidant system? This book has the answers, so keep reading.

Xenobiotics

As mentioned above, xenobiotics are foreign substances, which originate from outside the body's external sources in the environment. We breathe them in, digest them, or absorb them through our skin.

Regulatory agencies like the FDA are tasked with safeguarding public health. But loopholes in the system allow potentially harmful substances to enter the market unchecked. Manufacturers often determine the safety of their own products. The problem with this is that profits are often placed as a higher priority over people's health.

The United States Food and Drug Administration (FDA) allows a manufacturer to decide whether an ingredient is safe to consume. All the manufacturer must do is hire their own experts to claim that the substance "is not harmful under the intended conditions of use."[2] This is known as the GRAS (Generally Recognized as Safe) label. This then becomes the green light to start adding this substance to food products. If the FDA notes the GRAS label and raises a question about the ingredient, the manufacturers can withdraw the ingredient, or sometimes they can find their next loophole to continue to use the ingredient in food products.

Consider this:

In 1939, there were 32 active pesticide ingredients registered with the federal government. We now have more than 80,000 chemicals in our environment, from air pollutants, pesticides, plastics, phthalates, flame retardants, herbicides, heavy metals, and more, that are not approved by the FDA and affect our well-being.[3]

Clearly, we have a problem. Fatigue is the biggest complaint people have, and it's not due to age. There are people in their sixties traveling the world full of energy, and those in their forties barely getting out of bed. The problem is not aging—it's a toxic overload!

According to a survey by the American Gastroenterological Association, approximately 40 percent of Americans report that their daily lives are disrupted by digestive problems, like bloating and abdominal pain.[4] Every one of my clients suffers from some sort of digestive problem!

Some people are able to remove toxins from their bodies more easily than others. This may be due to their environment (also known as epigenetics) and genetics. Many of us can eat a small number of processed grains, sweeteners, and industrial seed oils, or have a glass of wine, and not be affected negatively. But that is not the case for all of us.

And even for those who can manage sufficiently, we all need to beware of what enters our bodies every day, over and over again. Whatever we inhale, ingest, and absorb into our skin eventually circulates within our bloodstream and may be stored in our bodies, causing harm. Cleaning products, mattresses, toothpaste, coffee, cosmetics, pesticides, and exhaust fumes (and more) expose us to thousands of chemicals daily. Eventually, the body can't keep up with being attacked by all these toxins and can't continue to protect us.

It's up to you to take responsibility, to take charge of your health. As you continue learning the facts, start asking questions. Be curious. Educate yourself. Buy products that support your health. This is your body, your life. You are in control.

The Connection Between Chronic Diseases and Toxins

From the moment we wake up to the time we return to our pillows to rest at night, we are bombarded with toxins. It's no wonder that nearly 95 percent of adults over the age of sixty have at least one chronic condition, according to the National Council on Aging (NCOA). Eighty percent have two or more chronic conditions, such as heart disease, arthritis, diabetes, and hypertension.[5]

Now counter these stats with this fact: These health conditions aren't a part of aging, even though we are taught to believe this. No, these conditions are due to the length of time we have allowed the toxins to accumulate in our bodies, without acknowledging and removing them.

Impaired functioning of our organs caused by chronic inflammation is where most diseases come from. And we, as stewards over our human bodies, create these diseases when we are chronically inflamed due to poor sleep, poor food choices, insufficient movement, and dwelling in our inner and outer toxic environments.

Through conventional medicine, we are being taught to treat diseases like type 2 diabetes with a pill. Doctors and pharmaceutical companies essentially look for the holes in our bodies and then provide a patch to put over those holes.

Most doctors are not equipped or financially motivated to help you prevent the holes from appearing in the first place. Or to stop them from reappearing once they have appeared. So with conventional medicine the story goes like this: The patient goes to the doctor because they have a symptom caused by chronic inflammation, such as high blood pressure.

The doctor reaches for their prescription pad and prescribes a blood pressure medication to suppress and shut down the symptom.

What is the drug doing? It is telling the brain to ignore the warning signs. The drug says to the body, "Stop creating inflammation. We don't want your message. It is not important." So, for a little while, the body stops sending the inflammation message. But the body still hurts. The toxins are still there. What happens next? Another cry for help is shared. But again, the brain is taught to stop the body from manifesting these cries.

Do you recognize the cycle? We try to solve our health problems through medicine designed to let us ignore the symptoms that are trying to tell us there is a problem that needs to be addressed. Unfortunately, we only end up with further problems because we haven't addressed the root issue. We never figured out where the leak was coming from, what caused it, and most importantly, how to fix it.

Address the Root Cause with Functional Medicine

Functional medicine asks, "Why is there pain and inflammation in the first place? What is my body trying to tell me?" Functional medicine looks at the origin and source of the dysfunction, proactively seeking to reverse or rebalance the overall system.

In the case of someone with high blood pressure, the dysfunction could be due to:

- Dehydration
- Alcohol overuse
- Chronic stress
- Poor eating habits

- Lack of nutrients
- Limited movement
- A disturbance in gut health
- A combination of several of these and other factors

Considering all these potential causes takes time and resources, right? And this is where the magic comes in! This is where we have a chance to create the dream life. When functional medicine looks at the body as a whole system, it starts to ask, "How do we create health?" By focusing on creating a healthy body, we examine the inner systems and organs that are crying for help. Now, the symptoms are finally being heard, which means they can start to go away because we found the problem. And the disease, as a side effect of all that was wrong inside, also goes away.

By understanding the true nature of biology, we discover a complex ecosystem—our bodies—that we have been blessed to care for! Our complex and marvelous bodies need to be in balance in order for us to be healthy. But when our bodies are out of balance, we get sick. It's really that simple.

Let's Check In

I realize we've covered a lot of complex information. I know this can feel overwhelming, but trust me: As you keep reading these pages, you'll gain more clarity and understanding. Take a break and gather your thoughts. In your health journal, write down answers to these questions:

- What have been the specific aha moments for you so far in reading this book?
- What do you think are the reasons for the symptoms you are experiencing?

- How does this knowledge influence how you look at your body and your responsibility to care for it?

Listen to Your Body

My husband and I recently traveled to Los Angeles for my daughter, Summer's, brain scans. Summer wasn't breathing when she was born and has struggled with numerous genetic polymorphisms—variations in genetic codes that affect how genes function and express themselves. These polymorphisms make it difficult for her body to remove toxins, which led to intrusive thoughts and facial tics as a teenager. Given my pharmaceutical background, I wanted to ensure her brain wasn't inflamed.

We chose to stay in Santa Monica for its convenient location close to the clinic. The moment I walked into our hotel room, I was hit by a musty smell emanating from the wall-to-wall carpeting. Why do beach hotels choose carpet, which is the perfect breeding ground for mold and moisture?

The first night was a nightmare. I wear a WHOOP Health Monitor on my wrist to measure my heart rate, sleep quality, and overall health. My heart rate variability (HRV) dropped from my usual fifties to the low twenties, and I felt like I'd been run over by a truck. HRV measures the variation in time between each heartbeat, reflecting the balance between your sympathetic (fight-or-flight) and parasympathetic (rest-and-digest) nervous systems. A low HRV indicates your body is under stress and not recovering well, triggered by toxins or stress.

I felt incredibly fatigued, had brain fog, and my whole body ached. After spending a few hours outdoors, my head started to clear. I took all my supplements—glutathione, NAC, glycine, and alpha-lipoic acid—to help remove the toxins my body had collected overnight.

We had to stay in the hotel two more nights. I was miserable but grateful I could feel the effects of toxicity. This experience taught me valuable lessons about making better choices when traveling.

The lesson: Pay attention to how you feel, whether you're at home or traveling. Don't ignore symptoms like headaches, low energy, and poor sleep—they're telling you something important. Take action—leave the area, ask for a different room, request an air filter, and take supplements to detox as much as you can. Listen to your body—it often knows more than we give it credit for.

Activity: Self-Assessment of Toxin Intake

Now that we know what toxins do to our bodies, it's time to get inspired to make the necessary changes. Although we can't heal our bodies overnight, we can identify the toxins that prevent us from being fully energized.

Grab a pen and paper and identify which of these statements you would answer "yes" to:

1. I wear perfume/cologne.
2. My home has wall-to-wall carpeting.
3. I've experienced a flood or roof, window, or pipe leak in the house or have visible water stains on the ceiling, walls, or window frames.
4. I regularly consume peanuts and corn.
5. I drink unfiltered tap water.
6. I consume water from plastic containers.
7. I cook with nonstick pots and pans, such as Teflon-coated cookware.

8. I use weed killers like Roundup in my yard.
9. I typically purchase conventional produce, meats, and poultry.
10. I use scented candles or air freshening products like plug-ins and sprays.
11. I enjoy a glass or two of wine every day.
12. I eat prepared food I buy in grocery stores most of the days of the week.
13. I eat in restaurants three or more times per week.
14. I use toothpaste with fluoride.
15. I am in a dysfunctional relationship and am constantly worried and fearful.

If you are overwhelmed by the number of *yes* answers you have, you are not alone. Fortunately, functional medicine can help. Awareness is the first step. Now that you know these are a potential source of toxins in your environment, the next step is to be inspired to change!

Identify Toxins

This section will go over some of the toxins we encounter in our daily life. Although you can't change your world overnight, you can continue to learn and make strategic changes one step at a time.

Here are three simple steps to creating good health when it comes to toxins.

Step 1: Identify

Identify which toxins may be affecting you in your everyday life.

Step 2: Remove

Remove these toxins from your environment, one at a time.

Step 3: Nourish

Fill your body with nutrients to support your detoxification pathways. Eat organic plants, high-quality protein, and healthy fats, and drink clean water. Healing can also be induced with better sleep, exercise, self-care, and fasting protocols.

Review and identify the list of toxins below that may be lurking in your environment and start to remove them one at a time. Additional steps will follow on how you can make simple and effective changes toward a healthier life.

Alcohol and Smoking

Let's be honest. Alcohol is poison to our livers and our bodies, despite the fact that we can keep drinking every day and continue to live. That shows the power of the incredible detoxification organ, the liver. Research consistently shows that even moderate alcohol consumption raises the risk of breast cancer.[6] There is no safe amount of smoking and alcohol.

Many of us like to enjoy a glass of wine, a beer, or a cocktail. Keep in mind, however, that alcohol is poison, and as is the case with any poison, whenever you drink it, the body's main priority is to remove it as fast as possible. This means that all the other important daily reactions to keep your body functioning and thriving are put on hold until the alcohol is removed. And when it comes to smoking, studies have shown that nicotine from cigarettes directly affects fat cells and alters them in such a way as to promote insulin resistance.

Sugar

Sugar should be part of an occasional dessert, not part of an everyday lifestyle. Unfortunately, sugar is everywhere. Fresh fruit juices, other sugary drinks, dried fruits, agave, corn syrup, dressings, sauces, fruit smoothies, ultraprocessed foods, and restaurant meals are all full of fructose, which causes inflammation. Even processed grains like pizza, pasta, and muffins act like sugar in the body because they are stripped of fiber and nutrients.

Lowering your sugar intake reduces the risk of many diseases.

While whole fruit is healthy, fruit juice is not. Whole fruit contains fiber that slows sugar absorption, while fruit juice causes a rapid spike in blood glucose, triggering large releases of insulin from your pancreas. Frequent insulin spikes lead to inflammation, artery damage, and various diseases.

Fructose is found in over 70 percent of processed foods under as many as 262 different names.[7] Unlike glucose, which is important in small amounts for energy, fructose actually depletes your energy. It also damages your gut-lining cells, allowing endotoxins—harmful substances released by bacteria—to enter the bloodstream and cause inflammation. Fructose is converted into glycerol in the liver, which is then used to turn free fatty acids into triglycerides (fat). The more fructose you consume, the more glycerol is available to create and store fat.

Metabolizing fructose results in waste products, including uric acid; excess uric acid can lead to high blood pressure and gout. Fructose is as addictive as alcohol and has no essential function in the body. It also increases hunger, leading to the overconsumption of empty calories and more fat storage.

Processed Seed Oils, Vegetable Oils, and Trans Fats

Avoid margarine, canola, cottonseed, corn, peanut (due to mold concerns), vegetable, grapeseed, soybean, sunflower, and safflower oils. These oils are chemically processed, bleached, and too high in omega-6 fatty acids, which are proinflammatory when coming from these processed sources. These oils are cheap, flavorless, and help preserve food; that is why they are commonly found in ultraprocessed foods, dressings, and restaurant meals.

Unfortunately, soybean oil, which is very high in omega-6 fatty acids, has become a significant component of the American diet over the past century.[8] While we do need some omega-6 fatty acids, they should come from whole foods like nuts, seeds, and chicken, not from chemically processed frying oils that cause inflammation and are associated with increased risks of various inflammatory diseases, including cardiovascular disease, metabolic syndrome, rheumatoid arthritis, asthma, cancer, and autoimmune diseases.[9]

Always avoid anything labeled "hydrogenated." Trans fats, another harmful ingredient to avoid, are created by adding extra hydrogen to vegetable oils to increase their shelf life. Although trans fats have been banned in many places, they can still be found in some ultraprocessed fast foods. Trans fats promote inflammation and damage cells.

Food Additives

Processed and ultraprocessed foods filled with flavorings, emulsifiers, and other chemicals cause DNA, intestinal, and neurological damage. While food additives prolong a product's shelf life, they shorten your life.

This is also the case for preservatives like colorings, artificial colors and flavors, and natural flavors like azodicarbonamide; butylated hydroxyanisole (BHA); butylated hydroxytoluene (BHT); calcium peroxide; calcium propionate; caramel coloring; carrageenan; cellulose; citric acid; sodium benzoate, nitrates and nitrites; and synthetic vitamins like folic acid, tert-butyl hydroquinone (TBHQ), titanium dioxide, and vanillin.

Fluoride

Fluoride is found in water, mouthwash, dental floss, and toothpaste. Studies have indicated a potential link between fluoride exposure and thyroid dysfunction, particularly hypothyroidism.

Mycotoxins and Mold

Mycotoxins can be found in peanuts, corn, grains, coffee, and our homes. They can cause symptoms like brain fog, allergies, chronic coughing, joint pain, and rashes, and can lead to cancer.

Antibiotics and Hormones

Antibiotics, by definition, disrupt the microbiome. And you don't have to take antibiotics to be at risk. The recombinant bovine growth hormone (rbGH) is a synthetic growth hormone injected into cows to increase milk production. This increases insulin-like growth factor 1 (IGF-1) in humans, which increases the risk of breast and prostate cancer. The rbGH in milk is similar in structure to insulin. It plays an important role in childhood growth and continues to have anabolic effects in adults. IGF-1 is stimulated by growth hormones (GH). It promotes cell growth and development in various tissues, including muscle and bone, and has significant effects on metabolism and cell repair. Elevated levels of IGF-1 have been linked to various conditions, including cancer and acromegaly, while low levels can result in growth deficiencies.[10]

What animals eat or are injected with, you eat.

There are situations where taking antibiotics is necessary, but the overuse of them can be damaging to our gut lining and kill beneficial gut bacteria as well as damage the protective lining of the gut.

Hormones and antibiotics, along with other pharmaceuticals, are also found in unfiltered tap water. They can enter our water supply through agricultural runoff and improper disposal of medications.

Pesticides, Insecticides, Herbicides

These are found in fruits, vegetables, and grains. Atrazine and glyphosate are the most commonly applied weed-control herbicides in the world. One widely used herbicide that causes oxidative stress is paraquat. It is highly toxic, yet still used in many herbicide brands due to its superior weed-control capabilities. These chemicals have permeated our air and water from the groundwater. They kill a lot of good bacteria! Essentially acting as antibiotics, these chemicals create holes in our gut lining and directly impact the microbiome by killing off your best friends. These chemicals bind to minerals from the food you eat so you can't absorb and use them.[11]

Parabens

Commonly found in cosmetics, shampoos, moisturizers, makeup, shaving cream, and in food as preservatives, parabens bind to hormone receptors, altering hormonal activity, and they directly impact the functions of our bodies They are linked to DNA damage, infertility, and many other health problems.[12]

Heavy Metals

Heavy metals like mercury can be found in large fish like tuna. Cadmium can be found in chocolate. Arsenic can be found in grains like rice, and lead can be found in water. Heavy metals are naturally occurring, but in high levels they will cause tissue damage.

Avoid eating large fish like tuna and swordfish. Look for organic, third-party-tested products if possible. For example, many chocolate companies are transparent about their lab tests for heavy metals on their website, and you can also email your favorite chocolate company and ask for the lab results. There are naturally occurring heavy metals in the soil, and our goal is to minimize our exposure to them, not to completely eliminate it. For rice, I'd suggest organic California rice, as it seems to contain the least amount of arsenic.

Increased Zonulin

Most of your immune system is in your gut. Gluten (the protein in wheat) increases zonulin production. Zonulin is a naturally occurring protein in your gut that regulates the permeability of the tight junctions between cells (the wooden fence) in the lining of the intestines. When zonulin production increases, these tight junctions loosen and increase intestinal permeability. This condition is often referred to as "leaky gut" and can lead to "leaky brain" syndrome.[13]

When the gut lining becomes damaged, the tight junctions loosen, allowing larger, undigested food particles, toxins, and bacteria to pass through the intestinal walls into the bloodstream. These substances, normally. contained within the gut, can then circulate throughout the body, potentially causing inflammation and affecting brain function. The immune system responds; it has to mark and remove these foreign objects, which is leading to systemic inflammation. This inflammation can contribute to various health issues, including autoimmune diseases, allergies, and chronic inflammatory conditions. It can also lead to nutrient deficiencies and malnutrition.[14]

High, Dry Heat in Cooking

The way we cook our food can produce pretty unhealthy results. Frying, charring, high, dry heat, and grilling create advanced glycation end products (AGEs) and acrylamide.

AGEs are compounds formed when proteins like collagen or fats combine with sugars in the bloodstream through a process called *glycation*. They contribute to the stiffening of the skin and other tissues by cross-linking collagen and elastin fibers. This process not only affects skin elasticity but also impacts blood vessels and heart tissue, potentially leading to cardiovascular issues. When you eat baked chicken that has been cooked at a high temperature, with that crispy skin, you are consuming AGEs, which makes your blood vessels crispy. That's not good.

Acrylamide is a chemical that can form in some foods during high-temperature cooking, particularly in common starchy foods like potatoes and bread. Acrylamide has been identified as a potential carcinogen.[15]

Also, high-heat, dry cooking creates toxic molecules that create reactive oxygen species (ROS) and cause cell death and organ damage.[16]

Triclosan

Triclosan can be found in antibacterial soaps, household cleaners, hand sanitizers, antibacterial cutting boards, and shower curtains. It is linked to hormone disruption, immune and thyroid impairment, and antibiotic resistance.[17] Triclosan also disrupts the gut microbiome.

Petrochemicals and plastics

Plastics are hormone disruptors. Research suggests that the estrogenic effects of bisphenol A (BPA) and other bisphenols found in plastic products like water bottles, food containers, and thermal receipts may cause insulin resistance by increasing insulin release from the pancreas.[18] BPA is just one type of petrochemical and a xenoestrogen that mimics estrogen and affects other hormones.

Plastic byproducts are also classified as obesogens, which interfere with fat cell growth and production. They increase the number and size of fat cells, contributing to weight gain.

A recent study highlighted the presence of nanoplastics in the bloodstream and their potential link to cardiovascular diseases, including heart attacks.[19]

Phthalates

Phthalates are found in anything with a fragrance. This includes:

- Perfume/cologne, shaving cream, hair styling products, makeup, sunscreens, food containers,

hair coloring, scented lotions, deodorants, and
menstrual pads.

- Fumes, candles, air fresheners, volatile chemical
products from paints and glues, paraquat (a pesticide), trichloroethylene (TCE), which is an industrial
solvent used in glues, carpet cleaners, paint remover,
metal degreasers, and dry cleaning. These are linked
to cancer[20] and Parkinson's disease, and they also
increase oxidative stress.[21]

Flame Retardants

Polybrominated diphenyl ethers (PBDEs) are flame retardants—compounds commonly applied to fabrics, carpets,
furniture, cell phones, and many other household items. New
evidence suggests that exposure to flame retardants more
than quadruples the risk of dying from cancer. PBDEs are
known as endocrine (hormone) disruptors. Anything that
disrupts the normal hormone function is going to cause
health problems.

Perfluoroalkyl and Polyfluoroalkyl Substances (PFAS)

Found in nonstick cookware, unfiltered water, food packaging like microwave popcorn bags, and the fabric of many
popular clothing brands, these "forever chemicals" do not
readily decompose and get excreted from our bodies. These
chemicals have been linked to mitochondria damage and
microbiome damage.[22]

Dry-Cleaned Clothes

Dry-cleaned clothes often retain chemical solvents like perchloroethylene, a known carcinogen.

Chronic Stress

Fear, worry, watching the news, and constant phone scrolling can cause chronic stress. This raises the level of the hormone cortisol, which then increases glucose production through a process called *gluconeogenesis*. Over time, this leads to chronic inflammation and disease in the gut, mitochondria, and the whole body.

Electromagnetic Fields (EMF)

EMFs, emitted from devices, are harmful because they are sticky. They adhere to cells, leading to inflammation.

Toss the AirPods and shut off your Wi-Fi at night while you sleep. These are two simple steps you can take now to reduce your exposure to EMFs and lower cell damage.

Sedentary Lifestyle

Inactivity can lead to chronic inflammation in the body. When we don't move enough, our muscles produce fewer anti-inflammatory proteins called myokines. While exercise temporarily increases inflammation as an adaptation mechanism to make you stronger, inactivity causes persistent inflammation, as indicated by elevated levels of C-reactive proteins (CRP). Regular movement helps push glucose from the blood into the cells, reducing blood sugar levels and inflammation. Without consistent activity, glucose remains in the bloodstream, contributing to ongoing inflammation.

Let's Pause

I can only assume that you might feel like everything around you is going to kill you. Take a deep breath. I know this can feel overwhelming. Yes, this is reality, but understanding it is the first step toward living well. So take a moment to let this information sink in. You don't need to memorize any of this; simply being aware is enough to start making better choices for yourself. Remember, every small change you make can lead to significant improvements. Every choice matters, and awareness is the first step. You've got this.

The Power of Renewal:
How Detoxification Can Transform Your Life

Jen, one of my dear clients, endured almost daily migraines, relentless bloating, and crushing fatigue. She believed, as many of my clients do, that she was eating "pretty healthy." But as we delved deeper, we uncovered hidden toxins in her daily life that were wreaking havoc on her body.

Plastic food containers and water bottles, Teflon pans, sugary conventional salad dressings, and prepared foods were silently loading her system with harmful substances every day. Determined to feel and function well, Jen made the shift quickly. She replaced plastic bottles with glass, discarded store-bought dressings, opted for healthier snacks, and brought her homemade meals to work.

The transformation was nothing short of miraculous. In just two short weeks, Jen's migraines vanished, and her persistent fatigue became a thing of the past. She felt full of life again.

Jen's story is a testament to the incredible changes that can happen when we are honest about our health and willing to make necessary adjustments. Her journey from suffering to thriving serves as an inspiration, reminding us all that with determination, support, and the right choices natural to our biology, we can overcome even the most daunting health challenges.

Our everyday decisions can lead to remarkable improvements in our well-being. By making small, consistent changes, we can transform our health and feel, function, and look the way we desire. We are supposed to feel great.

Detoxifying Is Often Misunderstood

Imagine if you take the trash out of your house once a year or vacuum once a year. When people hear "detox" or "cleanse," they often think of quick, short-term fixes. But detoxifying is a natural, ongoing process, much like sleep. Our bodies are constantly detoxifying, every minute of every day. To support this, we need to support the dream team, M&M, by eating fiber and polyphenol-rich foods.

Fiber helps by binding to toxins in the digestive tract, aiding their elimination. Polyphenols, powerful antioxidants found in colorful fruits, vegetables, and whole foods, combat oxidative stress and inflammation, supporting the body's natural detox processes.

Just like you regularly take out the trash at home, you need to eliminate waste from your body. The health of your detoxification system must be considered at all times. This involves cleansing the liver, kidneys, digestive tract, lungs, skin, and lymphatic system.

So, how do you detox? While a gentle cleanse might be beneficial after overindulging, most popularly promoted detoxes can do more harm than good. Because of this, it's essential to understand how detoxification works.

The body has an amazing capacity to process and dispose of toxins. But, like any waste-disposal system, it has limitations; the consequences can be hard when the body's capacity to process toxins is hindered. Impaired detoxification deprives the entire body of clean blood supply, and, consequently, every cell suffers. Toxins build up in tissues, slow down metabolism, and degrade health. Many of the toxic substances that enter the body are fat soluble, which means they dissolve only in fatty or oily solutions and not in water. This makes them difficult for the body to excrete. Toxins may be stored for years in fatty tissues, and are released during times of exercise, stress, or fasting. During the release of these toxins, symptoms such as headaches, brain fog, and low energy can manifest.

Detoxification happens in three phases, much like identifying, cleaning up, and taking out the trash at home. Here's a simplified explanation.

Phase 1—Identification: Spotting the Mess

Imagine this phase as identifying and sorting through all the trash in your house. You go through each room, identifying and breaking down the clutter into smaller, more manageable pieces, easier to carry out of the house (your body).

During this phase, the body identifies harmful substances mostly stored in our fat tissues and starts to release them from the fat and break them down into smaller, or different, molecules so they can be eliminated in the last phase. But the initial breakdown of toxins into intermediate forms can sometimes be more reactive or toxic than the original substances.

This process involves various chemical reactions that make the toxins easier to handle. Specialized enzymes known as the cytochromes P450 (CYPs) are a family of proteins that are the main elements in the liver responsible for the detoxification process, which means breaking down foreign substances like drugs and many other substances like our own hormones and cholesterol. These are extremely important proteins, and the activity of these enzymes (enzymes are made of proteins) can vary from person to person due to genetic differences (polymorphism), which is why a personalized approach to health is absolutely essential. If your function of CYPs is lower, you are not able to break down toxins as well as someone who is genetically predisposed to better function of CYPs. Also, many natural food substances may lower the function of CYPs.

Phase 2—Conjugation: Neutralization

Now we are bagging up the sorted trash and taking it out to the curb for collection.

In this phase, the body attaches water-soluble molecules to the reactive byproducts from phase 1, making them easier to eliminate.

The key water-soluble substances in the liver are glucuronic acid, sulfur, or amino acids (glutathione conjugates). Now the substances are neutralized, less toxic, and easier to eliminate.

Phase 3—Elimination: Taking out the Trash

The final phase involves the transport of these conjugated toxins out of the cells and into the bile and urine for excretion. We also eliminate toxins via sweat and breath. This phase relies on various transporter proteins to move the detoxified substances across cell membranes and out of the body, and requires good hydration, fiber, and a healthy microbiome. This is why it's important to have a healthy poop at least once every day! It's like taking the trash out.

As you can see, Phase 1 working well on its own is not enough. If you only sort the trash and don't take it out, your house will still be cluttered and stinky. Similarly, if the body only breaks down toxins without removing them, these intermediate substances will get reabsorbed and can be even more harmful than they were before they were broken down.

By understanding these phases, you can better appreciate how your body naturally detoxifies and understand the importance of supporting both phases of detoxification.

So how do you support all these detoxification pathways? The answer is simple: with real, whole organic foods and supplements, and movement:

- Cruciferous vegetables like broccoli, cauliflower, and brussels sprouts. These vegetables contain compounds like indole-3-carbinol, which can induce the production of cytochrome P450 enzymes.
- Citrus fruits and berries.
- Allium vegetables like onions and garlic.
- Nuts and seeds that are rich in vitamin E and magnesium.

- Physical activity, which can boost overall metabolic processes, including the activity of cytochrome P450 enzymes.
- Supplements like milk thistle, which contains silymarin. This enhances the activity of cytochrome P450 enzymes. N-acetylcysteine (NAC) is an antioxidant supplement that acts as a precursor to glutathione and supports detoxification pathways. Glutathione is a powerful antioxidant that helps neutralize toxins.
- B vitamins (B2, B3, B6, B12, methyl folate).

Create Your Strategy

It's evident that our surroundings are laden with toxic chemicals. From our food to our personal care products to even our thoughts, toxins infiltrate every aspect of our lives. This can feel overwhelming.

Take it one step at the time. Do a little bit today, then a little bit more next week. As you start to see results, you will build habits that will become a sustainable, healthy lifestyle. Keep in mind that every action we take has consequences, which means there is hope. By understanding the sources of toxins and implementing strategies to minimize their impact, we can live a strong, healthy life.

Success is achieved by taking consistent simple, achievable steps, one at a time.

Be Curious

Ask questions. When you are at the market and in the restaurant, ask if the produce is organic, if the fish is wild, if the meat is grass-fed and grass-finished. Are there added sugars? What oils are being used in the food you are about to buy?

Believe it or not, locally grown is not always the healthiest option. So just ask again and again.[23]

Read Ingredient Labels: It's Nonnegotiable

Every time you buy packaged food, get into the habit of reading ingredient labels. Ignore the front of the package, which is just pure marketing to entice you to buy the product; you don't get any useful, honest information there. Instead, always be sure to read the ingredients label on the back of the package. Watch out for all the toxins mentioned above, like added sugars, processed oils, and ingredients you can't recognize and don't have in your own kitchen. Download nutrition apps to help you decode the ingredients. A few good ones are Think Dirty, Healthy Living, or AskZoe.

Eat

Eat organic and in-season produce, regenerative-grown-and-raised food, wild or grass-fed, farm-raised animal protein, and wild, small seafood whenever possible.

Your nuts are best organic and sprouted. Enjoy chia, pumpkin, and hemp seeds.

Drink green tea if you can tolerate caffeine or go decaf and enjoy herbal teas.

Use organic oils and fats: extra virgin olive oil, avocado oil, macadamia oil, unrefined sesame oil, pumpkin seed oil, flaxseed oil, hemp oil, grass-fed organic butter, MCT oil, and coconut oil.

Always pay attention to how your unique biology responds to saturated and unsaturated fats.

Brew your organic, mold-free coffee in a glass French press.

Eat at home with fresh ingredients most of the time.

Eliminate canned food products, or make sure they do not contain BPA or its relatives in the lining.

Do not take paper receipts, which often contain BPA, at shops.

Hydrate

Adequate hydration is essential for supporting key pathways that expel toxins from the body. I start my day with about one liter of pure water every morning. Be sure to hydrate often with filtered water. Use a water filtration system like reverse osmosis, or search for reputable companies on the Environmental Working Group's website, ewg.org.

Monitor Sugar

Wear a continuous glucose monitor for at least one month to get to know your body. This tool will tell you how you respond to different kinds of carbohydrates in foods and will also provide plenty of resources and guidance.

Be Wise in Your Cooking

Replace nonstick toxic cookware with stainless steel or ceramic, carbon steel, cast iron, or enameled cast iron. Use stoneware for baking.

I also love my Vitaclay crock pot. I highly recommend it.

Eliminate Toxins Created by High Temperatures

Use lower-temperature cooking (320 degrees Fahrenheit and below) with higher moisture. Marinate food in acids like lemon juice and use herbs such as rosemary, oregano, and thyme to lower the formation of AGEs and acrylamids.

Try Smart Storage and Shopping

Buy products in glass jars as much as possible. Use reusable stainless, ceramic, or glass containers for your food and food on the go. Bring your own ceramic or stainless coffee mug into the coffee shop and use your glass, ceramic, or stainless-steel water bottles daily when leaving home.

Consider Your Clothes

Choose clothes made of untreated, natural materials such as unbleached cotton or hemp as much as possible. Find a cleaner that doesn't use toxic solvents. You can also air out your dry-cleaned clothes before bringing them into your house.

Upgrade Your Hygiene

Get fluoride-free toothpaste. Boka, Wellnesse, RiseWell, or Auromere are my favorites.

Replace your deodorant with a nontoxic, aluminum-free version.

Talk to your dentist about sealants and composites, which often contain BPA.

Make Your Home a Safe Sanctuary

Take your shoes off outside the door.

Use fragrance-free cleaning and laundry products. I love Branch Basics. There are many other companies making great laundry detergent products now.

Use unscented wool balls instead of dryer sheets.

Use essential oils, diffusers, and salt lamps instead of scented candles.

Be sure your mattress and bedding are organic, and made of natural products without fire retardants.

Filter your shower water with a whole-house filter or attached showerhead filter.

Get an air filter for your home, unless you are fortunate to live in the woods.

Additional Steps

Practice time-restricted eating (TRE), which means eating all your meals within an eight-to-ten-hour window and fasting (not eating) for fourteen to sixteen hours overnight each day. This helps optimize your digestive system and metabolic health, lowers inflammation, and gives the body the opportunity to focus on clearing out waste from the body instead of digesting food.

Get seven to nine hours of quality sleep every night.

Use near-infrared light therapy to promote cellular healing if you have access to it.

Methods for Detoxification
Touch the Ground Every Day

Grounding, also known as earthing, is the practice of connecting with the earth's surface to benefit and energize the body by collecting free electrons. When we touch the earth through our bare hands and feet, which have eccrine sweat glands, we absorb these beneficial free electrons that help balance our body's electrical charge. Here is how you benefit: mitigated negative effects of modern electromagnetic fields (EMFs), increased mitochondrial efficiency, improved cellular hydration, reduced systemic inflammation, decreased pain sensations, enhanced blood flow and circulation, normalized cortisol and stress responses, and better sleep quality.

Sweat It Out

Sweating is one of the most effective ways to detox, since many toxic elements are preferentially excreted through sweat. Studies have shown that sauna use is particularly effective at promoting the excretion of heavy metals, which may be a reason why frequent sauna use is associated with a reduced risk of death from cardiovascular disease.[24] Sweating also increases circulation and body heat, which helps in the transport and elimination of toxins through the liver and kidneys. Sauna use can also lower the amount of polybrominated diphenyl ethers (PBDEs) in the body, so it may also reduce risk of cancer.[25] PBDE is a class of flame-retardant chemicals used in many products, such as electronics, furniture, and textiles, to reduce the risk of fire.

Lymph Drainage

Schedule a massage, do regular dry brushing (you can find many resources online), and move a lot. Skipping or trampoline jumping daily is a great way to move the lymph system to remove the toxins.

Attend to Your Heart

Remember that your thoughts can also be toxic. Accordingly, identify those daily stressors that are triggers and replace them with gratitude-filled thoughts.

The goal is to create a healthy environment within all aspects of your life. We will go deep into this in the chapter on inner environment and transformation.

Until then, do at least one thing every day that makes you happy. Dance, draw, walk your dogs, journal—anything that fills your heart with love.

Action Plan

1. Select one thing from these detoxification ideas that you will incorporate into your day or week.
2. Write it down in your health journal.
3. Share this goal with a family member or friend who will help keep you accountable.

Detoxification Is a Lifestyle, Not an Event

In this chapter you learned that we are always detoxifying, twenty-four hours a day, seven days a week. We are exposed to toxins daily and create toxic byproducts from our own energy production.

We want to build a mindset of detoxifying every day.

The best way to minimize toxins is to first identify the toxins in your life. Then modify your lifestyle to reduce or eliminate exposure to them, and nourish your body. It's that simple.

You now understand how to identify and eliminate toxins, so you can create a strategy for doing this, which is your first step toward better health. Bit by bit, you will be adding to this strategy. You will be amazed how just a shift in mindset will create a shift in your health. More and more, you will feel empowered. And the more you learn, the more you will be able to cultivate a life of greater health.

Lab Tests

If you're considering delving deeper into understanding your own health and potential toxic load, various lab tests can provide valuable insights. It's essential to work with a knowledgeable functional medicine doctor to interpret these results and guide you through incorporating your response to them into your lifestyle. You can find reputable practitioners through resources like the Institute for Functional Medicine's practitioner directory at https://www.ifm.org/find-a-practitioner.

- **Genetic Testing: Personalize Your Life**
  A good place to start may be genetic testing to determine how well you detoxify based on your genetics, so you can support your body better with your lifestyle.

  Talk to your functional medicine practitioner about these tests. I like to use 3X4 Genetics and StrateGene genetic tests.

- **Alzheimer's Risk Assessment**
  Consider adding an apolipoprotein E (ApoE) genotype test to your blood panel to assess your risk for Alzheimer's disease, to again create a lifestyle supporting your health.

- **Toxic Load Assessment**

Explore tests such as the organic acids test, heavy metals analysis (like Genova Diagnostics or Quicksilver Scientific Heavy Metal testing), and the DUTCH Test to evaluate estrogen metabolism and toxic pathways that may lead to various health issues, including cancer.

- **Mold Exposure Screening**
  If you're concerned about mold exposure, try a myco-toxin test like the Mycotox test from Mosaic Diagnostics.
- **Infection Detection**
  Tests such as ParaWellness can identify viruses, parasites, bacteria, and yeast that may be impacting your health.
- **Inflammation Monitoring**
  Keep track of your inflammation levels with tests like high-sensitivity C-reactive-protein (hsCRP), fasting insulin, blood glucose or HbA1c, fibrinogen, uric acid, homocysteine, insulin, iron, gamma-glutamyl trans-ferase (GGT) in your liver, and lipid peroxidation. These markers provide insights into inflammation, oxidative stress, and metabolic health.

By investing in these tests, you gain valuable insights into your health status and can tailor your lifestyle choices accordingly to optimize your life. Investing in your health now can save you from potential medical expenses and complications in the future.

Prioritize spending on health maintenance rather than disease management.

This chapter has covered a lot information on toxins—what they are, how they impact your health, and the crucial steps you can take to reduce exposure to them. From understanding the sources of toxins in your environment to supporting your body's natural detoxification systems, each section provides actionable insights designed to help you create a healthier life.

Health is an ongoing journey, and this chapter is meant to be a resource you return to whenever you need guidance, a reminder, or clarity. Let this chapter serve as your go-to reference. As you continue to make small, consistent changes, know that you are building a stronger foundation for your long-term vibrant health.

CHAPTER TWO

THE POWER OF REAL, WHOLE FOODS

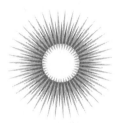

The Power of Real, Whole Foods

As a young adult, Sara already was suffering from debilitating migraines and persistent stomach pains. Seeking relief, she visited clinic after clinic, where doctors prescribed medications to give her temporary relief but failed to address the root cause of her issues. Over time, the medications became less effective, and Sara's health continued to decline.

Like many, Sara grew up with a "no limits" philosophy around food—embracing fried foods, chips, sodas, chocolate, cakes, cookies, muffins, and eating out. In her perception, these weren't unhealthy processed foods; they were simply what she enjoyed eating. Sara's seemingly harmless dietary habits, lack of an exercise routine, and late nights eventually caught up with her.

Her breaking point came when the pain became unbearable, prompting her to seek a lasting solution. That's when she reached out to me, ready for change but uncertain where to begin.

Our journey started with unraveling Sara's eating habits and sleep routine. Understanding the impact of her food choices and rest was foundational to her health. We began with small, manageable changes, starting by identifying the toxins in her daily life. We focused on balancing her meals with lean proteins, healthy fats, and abundant vegetables, while eliminating the major culprits: alcohol, fried foods, and added sugars.

The goal wasn't restriction but transformation—replacing foods that exacerbated her symptoms with whole, nourishing foods that would heal her body from within. We created simple bedtime and morning routines to help her nervous system become more resilient.

As Sara embraced these changes, a remarkable transformation unfolded. Her migraines became less frequent and less severe, and her intestinal pains gradually subsided. More importantly, she gained an understanding of the fundamentals of her body, and regained control over her health after years of uncertainty and overwhelm. Understanding the profound connection between food, sleep, and well-being empowered Sara to make informed choices that supported her overall health.

Through this journey, Sara discovered that embracing a nutritionally balanced diet wasn't about deprivation; it was about liberation—nourishing her mind, body, and soul with foods that supported her well-being.

"I'm Really Struggling to Find a Diet That Works for Me."

This sentiment breaks my heart. I hear it almost every time I start working with someone who has been suffering with headaches, gut issues, pain, and extra weight. Desperate to feel better, they eliminate gluten, dairy, or other strategies they're exposed to on social media or the "search engine doctor." But they rarely succeed long-term.

We need to understand, as we covered in the previous chapter on toxins, that there is a lot more to proper nutrition than meets the eye. It's not just removing gluten and dairy from your diet. Developing a sound nutrition plan takes patient work; it won't happen in a week. Think about it: It took years to develop pain and discomfort, so it will take time to rebuild your body.

We just need to understand the simple fundamentals of our biology and food. Or rather, of how to nourish our bodies.

What Is Food, Really?

According to the Centers for Disease Control and Prevention (CDC), over ninety-eight million American adults have prediabetes, which is one in three adults, with approximately 80 percent unaware of their condition.[26] Prediabetes is a serious and potentially dangerous health condition that, if left untreated, significantly increases the risk of developing type 2 diabetes, heart disease, stroke, and various other conditions. These include nonalcoholic fatty liver disease, kidney disease, nerve damage (neuropathy), retinopathy leading to vision problems, and an elevated risk of certain cancers, such as breast and colon cancer.

Our progress over the years has led to some amazing technological advancements, especially in the food industry. As we evolved, so did our food processing techniques.

Today, it can be challenging to determine what is real food and what is processed and ultraprocessed food, and when processed foods become unhealthy. Not all processed foods are bad. They exist on a spectrum, and understanding this spectrum is crucial.

Let's start by clarifying the difference between processed and ultraprocessed factory foods. The US Department of Agriculture defines *processed foods* as those that have undergone any changes from their natural state. This includes actions like washing, cleaning, fermenting, freezing, heating, chopping, pasteurizing, canning, and packaging. It can also involve adding preservatives, flavors, and many other additives.[27]

Many processing techniques offer benefits in terms of convenience and health. Processed food is any food that has been altered in some way from its natural state, usually for safety reasons or convenience. It's the amount and type of processing that matters.

For example, hard-boiled eggs, fruits and vegetables frozen to extend shelf life and reduce food waste, and fermented foods like yogurt, kimchi, and kombucha are all processed foods, and understandably healthy.

On the other hand, ultraprocessed foods (UPFs) take processing to a whole other level. These foods are industrial formulations made primarily or entirely from extracted substances derived from foods. They often contain added processed starches, sugars, hydrogenated oils, and a very long list of additives, artificial flavors, emulsifiers, and other preservatives, as mentioned in the previous chapter on toxins. Ultraprocessed foods are a bit of a trap in that they're often designed to be highly palatable and ultraconvenient. This combination makes them a more tempting option than more nutritious and filling real, whole foods.

Ultraprocessed foods like soda and energy drinks, packaged snacks such as protein bars, chips and cookies, frozen meals, microwavable dinners, and processed meats like hot dogs and deli meats are highly palatable and convenient, though they're often missing or are low in essential nutrients, and they contain unrecognizable ingredients.

Have you ever wondered how it's possible for the bread in grocery stores to sit on the shelves for days and not change its structure, smell, or color?

Many people think that as long as food doesn't come from a fast-food place, it is "pretty" healthy. Unfortunately, that is not the case. Ultraprocessed food can also be found in grocery stores and restaurants. This category of food is not just processed; it is significantly altered from its original form—your body does not recognize it and cannot create energy and build a strong body from it. The body actually sees it as a foreign object that needs to be fought against. It damages you on every level. Do you remember your precious dream team, M&M? UPF (ultraprocessed food) damages them.

Eating at restaurants and consuming premade grocery-store meals can be just as harmful as frequenting fast-food drive-throughs. Restaurant meals and premade foods often contain hidden additives, sugars, MSG, flavorings, mold, preservatives, unhealthy fats, and flavorings. These ingredients can wreak havoc on your gut microbiome and mitochondria, leading to chronic inflammation and a host of other health issues like fatigue, bloating, and headaches.

Unfortunately, unless the substance we eat kills us immediately, we call anything we put into our mouth "food." How about those substances that are slowly killing us? Like the potatoes fried in soybean oil, chips, frozen dinners with a bunch of additives that are wrapped in plastic containers, protein bars with sugar and artificial flavorings, and salad dressings with emulsifiers.

You may be thinking you eat healthy, just like the majority of my clients and friends believe—until they understand the differences between real foods and UPFs and recognize the effects they have on our bodies.

Are you eating "healthy" foods? Let's be honest. Look at everything you put in your mouth. Does your daily food come out of bags and boxes, or can you classify it as real, whole foods? For a helpful list of food terms, see the glossary at the end of this chapter.

Real, Whole Foods

You will hear me talk about real food in this book. When I think of real, whole foods, I think of food from healthy organic fields, not factories. It's a substance that is as close to nature as possible. Real food gives us energy and the building blocks to grow and repair. It is what M&M need to create energy for us to live well.

The closer the food is to nature, the closer it is to your health. Repeat: *The closer the food is to nature, the closure it is to your health.*

When you think about real food as a nutritional substance that is supposed to provide building blocks for growth and repair, and energy, you do not need to worry about "diets." Instead, think of real, whole foods that are not processed, like apples, or minimally processed, like cooked beans, eggs, yogurt, or wild meat, preferably processed in your home where you have control over all the ingredients going into the processing of the food.

What you decide to eat shapes your days, and in turn your entire life. Your choices make the difference between a thriving life and a life filled with headaches, pain, low energy, and dependency on medication.

That's why you need to think of food as more than just getting rid of hunger.

Living in the victim mindset, blaming genes, age, and other unrelated factors for proper health, is not helping us. You can take charge of your body—and of your life. I've seen countless clients become the people they want to be when they're honest with themselves. That's the first step we have to take.

I know food can be a complex, highly emotional topic. It's often hard to speak about with friends or family because it is so specific to each person's culture, environment, beliefs, and habits. Yet we must talk about food choices because they're the culprit of so many diseases and ailments. We need to compassionately and patiently address each of the issues that lead us to poor health. Thankfully, making small changes in your eating habits today can prevent chronic illness tomorrow.

Ask These Questions When Buying Food:
- How close is this substance to its natural form?
- How much processing did the food go through?

- What type of processing did it go through?
- What additives are included to increase its shelf life? The longer the shelf life, the shorter your life.
- What is the food packaged in? Is it packaged in plastic or metal or in paper with plastic lining?
- How is this food going to affect me today—and in the long term—based on my health and life goals?

Food Is Personal

The more you understand food, your environment, and yourself, the more you can be in charge and create the health you want. And that looks different for each of us—which is why you must be open-minded and willing to listen to your unique body.

We're overloaded with so many diet options, like paleo, which includes just meat and vegetables; and keto, which is just fat and a little bit of protein with very restricted carbohydrates. Mediterranean focuses on lots of plants, fish, and some meat. Then you have vegetarian and vegan, and so many more.

You have to know which foods work best for you at your stage of life. As we evolve, our environments change, our microbiomes change, and our needs change. These constant changes are based on many factors like age, environment, stress levels, exercise level, and more, so sticking to one way of eating every single day of your life is not sustainable. What you ate in your twenties may not work for you in your forties; that's the reality of biology. And this is especially true for women, who go through more drastic hormonal changes.

We all have unique responses to specific foods. Some of the factors that affect our reactions to foods include genetics, current energy level, current toxic load, current stress level, current physical health, current microbiome, current environment, and gender.

This is why testing is vital. You simply don't know what you can't measure. It can take years for symptoms from poor eating habits to develop; we may be eating food that harms us in the long run. How do you really know if what you are eating is working for your biology today and long-term? It's just a good idea to get to know your body through data, to learn how you respond to certain foods, and to see what deficiencies you may have due to genetics, stress, and other factors.

For example, if I didn't wear a CGM (continuous glucose monitor), I wouldn't know that my body doesn't respond well to sweet potatoes. They spike my glucose more than chocolate. I can also feel it because I feel hungry and sluggish after I eat them. I tried to eat them with loads of fat, protein, and fiber, but my body just does not react well to them. Once I saw the results on my glucose monitor, I connected the dots and stopped eating sweet potatoes in order to maintain my metabolic health. Meanwhile, when my husband eats sweet potatoes, his glucose stays stable.

There is no universal nutritional plan that works for every single person. That said, all of us need to consume the basic nutrients to be able to build tissue, muscle, bones, enzymes, and hormones, and to strengthen our immune system.

What to Test

Here are examples of what I test for my own health.

1. **I test my genetic profile.** As mentioned in the previous chapter, genetic testing helps me understand my predispositions and how I metabolize different foods. By knowing my genetic makeup, I gain insight into how my body functions and what specific needs it has. This knowledge allows me to tailor my environment and lifestyle to support my body optimally; it helps me make informed decisions about nutrition, exercise, and other lifestyle factors, ensuring I can create the best conditions for my health and well-being.

   We can't change our genes, but we can change our environment to influence our genes, and this is called epigenetics (*epi* means "above"—in this case, "above genes").

2. **I wear a continuous glucose monitor (CGM).** I recommend that my clients wear a CGM for at least one month, which is the minimum amount of time. This one tool can save your life, and it helps you discover how your body responds to food. This tool allows me to track everything I eat, and I can make additional notes about how I feel after I eat certain foods.

3. **I get a DEXA scan.** I measure my visceral fat, which is the fat around organs such as the heart, liver, and kidneys. The "silent killer" is the fat you can't see—this causes inflammation and disease. Go online and look for locations in your area to get a DEXA scan, and make sure to ask for bone, muscle, and fat measurements. It's an easy, low-radiation, quick, and reliable test that can give you truly lifesaving information.

4. **I measure my macro and micronutrients' digestion and absorption.** It's not just about what you eat, but what you digest and absorb. You can eat the best, real foods, but if your gut microbiome is not strong and healthy, and if your digestion doesn't work properly, you cannot break down the food and use the nutrients. I order a stool GI test and an organic acid test for myself and my clients, which you can ask your functional medicine doctor or other practitioner to do for you. These tests show the health of your microbiome and mitochondria. You can do this simple, noninvasive test from the comfort of your home.

Unraveling the Mystery: My Daughter's Journey to Health

My daughter Summer was just six years old when she noticed overly dry skin on her hands. Two fingers on one of her hands became so dry, they were red, itchy, flaky, and bleeding. It was evident there was inflammation in her body, but the source remained a mystery.

Despite what I believed to be a healthy lifestyle, the redness and itching gradually expanded, covering Summer's hands, body, and face with flaky, red spots. I tried various remedies, from oat baths to ghee butter, and covered her hands with bamboo gloves to retain moisture so she could sleep. Deep down, I knew the issue was internal. Her body was screaming for help, but I had no idea what to do.

Summer's pain and incessant itching disrupted her sleep, and I, too, couldn't sleep. Many nights I spent on the computer, searching helplessly for a clue to solve the issue. I researched doctors, nutritionists, specialists, and energy healers. I scoured PubMed for studies on similar cases, all in vain. Dermatologists prescribed hormone creams, which I never gave her. Not knowing the cause, I feared the creams might make her situation worse.

A food allergy test revealed Summer was allergic to almost everything, prompting me to explore restrictive diets—no eggs, dairy, or gluten—but still there were no improvements. I felt isolated in my efforts. Despite all my attempts, things only worsened, leaving me scared and emotionally drained. My days became consumed with thoughts of what more I could do and who else I could consult. This effort became my full-time job.

The turning point in Summer's story came when, drawing upon my education in pharmacy and functional medicine, I rejected conventional medications and persisted in searching for the root cause. After two years of relentless pursuit, we found hope at Dr. Mark Hyman's clinic, The UltraWellness Center, in Lenox, Massachusetts.

Through genetic testing and in-depth analyses, we uncovered that Summer struggled with detoxification due to multiple genetic mutations, which was leading to poor methylation and glutathione production, high fat absorption, lower insulin sensitivity, histamine intolerance, and difficulty removing dopamine and adrenaline. Understanding these genetic polymorphisms explained her struggles.

Despite the challenges, we embraced a lifestyle tailored to her needs, incorporating clean, organic food and daily supplements. Summer's inability to break down histamine and produce enough essential antioxidants posed ongoing challenges, but understanding the genetic basis of her issues gave me peace and allowed us to manage her condition effectively.

Today, as a teenager, Summer adheres to a lifestyle plan encompassing food, sleep, exercise, and her inner and outer environment. Witnessing the remarkable changes that occurred when we provided her body with what it uniquely required was both reassuring and empowering. We have created a lifestyle that works for Summer, allowing her to thrive.

While Summer is dependent on a few daily supplements for the rest of her life, and navigating adolescence presents its own set of challenges, I have simplified her diet and made it manageable. Her genetic makeup poses certain limitations, but I believe that genes are merely a loaded gun. The trigger gets pulled through the Standard American Diet (SAD), mold, other toxins, and chronic stress.

For Summer, it was remarkable to see the change that happened quickly once we gave her body what it needed. This is what's amazing about the human body! Our needs are unique, and one plan does not fit all. Once I created a lifestyle that worked for Summer's needs, she had the chance to thrive.

One universal truth for all of us is that removing toxins and living the lowest-toxin lifestyle possible ensures that you can rebuild your body and have an amazing and productive life. No matter what your increased risks are, the principles are the same: identify and eliminate toxic exposure, and nourish your body with real food. Summer's needs are higher than most and require constant adjustment of her supplements based on stress from school, traveling, and other normal routines, but the focus on real food remains paramount.

Ninety-eight percent of genetic polymorphisms do not cause diseases; what does is how you communicate with the genes, and food is one of the major communicators.[28] It's not the keys on the piano (the genes) that determine health; it's how you play the piano (food, sleep, inner environment, and movement) that determines the quality of your life.

The Importance of Protein

Every single bite of food that enters our mouths affects our health, either positively or negatively. So, when you eat real food, you're performing an act of self-love. And consuming protein is one of the best ways to be good to yourself. In fact, you are literally a pile of protein. If you don't eat protein, you don't exist.

Proteins are like a beautiful necklace made of beads, with amino acids being the beads themselves. Just as beads come together to form a necklace, amino acids are used in our bodies as building materials for muscles, tissues, joints, hormone synthesis, enzyme production, immune function, energy production, and so much more. There are twenty different amino acids, like beads of different shapes and colors, which come together to create unique proteins and other essential molecules necessary for life. These amino acids are categorized into nine essential ones, which we must obtain from our diet, and eleven nonessential ones, which the body can produce on its own.

The body cannot make the essential amino acids but can make the nonessential amino acids. But I would argue they are all essential, because you cannot make a protein without all twenty amino acids, and we are often deficient in all twenty. Biologists suggest there are at least ten thousand different types of proteins, based on the unique order of amino acids and protein foldings.[29]

To illustrate the importance of amino acids, let's look at three examples:

- *Tryptophan* is an important amino acid for the production of serotonin, which regulates mood and appetite. Serotonin is then metabolized into melatonin, which is the hormone we need to fall asleep. Without sufficient tryptophan, you might experience mood disorders like depression and insomnia due to low serotonin and melatonin levels.

- *Glutathione* molecules are made of the amino acids cysteine, glutamic, and glycine. Glutathione is the most important antioxidant made in the liver. It protects us from all oxidative stress and helps with detoxification. If glutathione levels drop, cells can die, leading to increased oxidative damage and a higher risk of chronic diseases like liver disease and cancer.

- *Methionine* is an amino acid crucial for the methylation process, a fundamental biochemical process that involves adding a methyl group (CH_3) to many molecules like DNA, proteins, and other substances, which is essential for DNA repair, detoxification, and overall health. The methylation process occurs billions of times every second. Without adequate methionine, you could suffer from impaired DNA repair and detoxification processes, leading to an increased risk of conditions like cardiovascular disease and cognitive decline.

Understanding Collagen Is More Important Than You Realize

Collagen is a type of protein crucial for the body's connective tissues. Historically, we used to consume animals from nose to tail and pick fresh berries and other plants rich in vitamin C and nutrients, which supported collagen production. Collagen is a peptide, meaning it's a smaller protein.

Collagen has a unique amino acid composition compared to other proteins, with uniquely high amounts of the amino acids proline, glycine, and hydroxyproline. Collagen is vital for creating and repairing all connective tissues, acting as the glue that holds everything together. It's essential for cardiovascular and joint health, as well as for healthy skin, hair, and nails.

Although the body can produce collagen, it needs the right micronutrients to do so efficiently. Vitamin C and the amino acids mentioned above are necessary for collagen synthesis. If you're experiencing tissue damage, joint pain, or ligament issues, I recommend increasing your daily intake of collagen to support repair and maintenance.

Muscles: The Largest Reservoirs of Protein in the Body

We do not store protein as we do fat and sugar. Your body relies on getting a regular supply of amino acids from food daily. If you do not eat enough protein regularly, the body goes to the existing muscle to get it. That's not good! Look what happens with many elderly people—they eat less food, especially protein, and start becoming frail.

It's important to understand that the goal isn't necessarily just to eat enough protein; it's a little bit more complex. It's about having adequate amounts of B vitamins and other micronutrients, as well as having a healthy gut microbiome and gut lining. A healthy digestive tract and adequate stomach acid are crucial for breaking down protein into amino acids. After proteins are broken down into amino acids, they become building blocks for what the body needs to make, from hormones, enzymes, and antioxidants like glutathione, to antibodies for the immune system. And that's why you need sufficient amounts of protein and a healthy gut to digest the protein efficiently.

How do you determine how much protein you need each day? The exact amount of protein you need depends on various factors such as your age, weight, activity level, gender, and stress level. Studies show that the optimal amount of protein is within the range of 1.2 to 1.6 grams per kilogram of body weight per day, which is about 0.8 grams per pound of body weight.[30]

Here's a step-by-step guide to help you calculate your daily protein needs and figure out how to split it into three meals:

1. *Convert your weight to kilograms* by dividing your weight in pounds by 2.2. Example: If you weigh 165 pounds, divide 165 by 2.2 to get approximately 75 kilograms, or go online and use a kilograms calculator.

2. *Multiply your weight in kilograms by 1.2* to find the lower end of your protein range. An example:

   75 kg x 1.2 g/kg = 90 grams of protein per day

3. *Divide the total daily protein requirement by 3* to evenly distribute your protein intake throughout the day:

90 grams of protein a day / 3 = 30 grams of
protein per meal, if you eat 3 times a day

Here are some examples of sources for about 30 grams of protein:
- 5 eggs
- 1 ½ cups yogurt
- 5 oz chicken breast
- 4 oz lean beef
- 6 oz salmon
- 24 oz bone broth
- 4 oz dry lupini pasta
- 3.5 oz lupini beans
- 1.75 cups lentils, cooked
- 3.75 cups quinoa, cooked
- 5 oz almonds
- 9 tbsp hemp seeds
- 2 cups black beans

Tip: Download my recipes on my website (they all have about 30 grams of protein):
https://yourwellness-madesimple.com/shop/.

Can Plants Supply Enough Protein?

Plant-based diets are popular, and for good reason. Plant fibers and nutrients are important for our overall health. The problem, however, is that when eating only plants, you won't get the right balance of amino acids. As such, you will need to eat more calories than if you ate meat and fish to get the amount of protein your body needs. This may be fine if you are an active person, though the extra calories to reach the protein goals may cause some problems for people who are more sedentary. There is also the option for supplementing with amino acids, though it's always best to get as many nutrients as possible from whole foods.

Important to know:
Legumes are deficient in the amino acid methionine, which is crucial for DNA protection and detoxification. This serves as an example for why eating a variety of foods is important.

Unless you're a strict vegan or vegetarian, consider these protein sources:
- 100% grass-fed and grass-finished meat
- Wild meat
- Wild, cold-water small fish: wild salmon, herring, sardines, anchovies
- Pasture-raised poultry
- Organic dairy and eggs

Focus on Quality

Food can get pretty expensive. With all our financial obligations, we have to make decisions on how much—or how little—we will spend on groceries.

That's understandable. Still, as best as you can, don't sacrifice quality for the sake of saving money. Our mitochondria and microbiome rely on nutritious food.

Conventional meats come from animals fed GMO corn and grains treated with pesticides, and injected with hormones and antibiotics, which are stored in the animal's fat. They are raised in an unhealthy, stressful environment, where they can easily become sick. You end up eating what the animal eats and is injected with. By buying grass-fed and wild meat, you support humanely raised animals, the environment, and yourself. This is one way to do some self-love and nature-love.

Fat Is Good for You

Contrary to popular belief, fat (healthy fat, that is) is an essential part of our healthy lifestyle.

- Our cell membranes are made of fat.
- Myelin, which aids in the protection of neurons, is made of fat.
- The brain, which is 60 percent fat, is completely dependent on high-quality fats. Fat is critical for happiness, memory, cognition, and learning, and regulates your mood and behavior.[31]
- Studies link a deficiency of omega-3 fatty acids to depression, anxiety, bipolar disorder, schizophrenia, and even violence.[32]
- Hormone production relies on fat.
- Fat is a clean energy source for exercise.
- Fat helps to slow our digestion, keeps us full longer, and prevents us from overeating.
- Fat is necessary to absorb fat-soluble vitamins like A, D, E, and K.

All Fat Is Not Created Equal

There has been a years-long debate in the health and wellness community about whether to eat saturated or unsaturated fats. To understand what to choose, we first have to under-stand a few quick facts.

Saturated fats are made of single bonds that stack together tightly, making them more stable, more resistant to heat, and less reactive, which make them less likely to oxidize. We already know that oxidation produces harmful chemicals like free radicals that cause inflammation, which can lead to many diseases. Saturated fats can be found in butter, lard, coconut oil, and ghee (clarified butter).

Unsaturated fats, such as monounsaturated and polyun-saturated fats, are liquid oils made up of double bonds that do not stack together tightly. They are sensitive to light and heat, making them more likely to oxidize. Examples include avocado oil, olive oil, fish oil, and pumpkin seed oil. For optimal health benefits, these oils are generally best used unheated, although using olive oil at low temperatures is okay.

To know which fat type to consume and cook with, I suggest you test and focus on how you feel after you use different types of quality fats. As long as you focus on quality, both types can be healthy options.

The right fats depend on each person. As for me, I can't tolerate saturated fats well; I get constipated and bloated. I also know I have a genetic predisposition that makes it hard for me to eliminate saturated fats. I stay away from coconut oil and butter for the most part and focus mainly on unsatu-rated healthy fats like olive oil or avocado oil. I also get daily fats from whole seeds and nuts, as well as fish and eggs.

How to Find Quality Fats

The best sources of fat are minimally processed as close to nature as possible. Those include:

- Olive oil and olives
- Avocado oil and avocados
- Eggs
- Sea vegetables such nori, kombu, and many others
- Nuts and seeds (sprouted, organic, and raw)
- Grass-fed and grass-finished meats
- Ghee butter (clarified butter)
- Butter
- Coconut oil
- Small cold-water fish like wild-caught salmon, sardines, anchovies, and herring. These contain omega-3 fatty acids, which are proven to reduce inflammation.[33] This is why higher blood levels are associated with a lower risk of heart attack, stroke, and Alzheimer's disease. Omega-3 fats make blood more slippery, reducing artery disease. They are also incredible for your brain health.

Tips for Quality Olive Oil

Olive oil is perhaps the most studied oil of all fats. It's high in antioxidants and polyphenols, and it's easy to use in both vegan or meat-based diets. When choosing your olive oil, follow these guidelines:

- Buy organic, cold-pressed oil in a dark glass bottle, which will lower the amount of oxidation.

- Try buying directly from a producer rather than a grocery store. This lowers the chances of the oil being oxidized by sitting on the shelf for long periods of time. Plus, it's difficult to be certain if olive oil in grocery stores is truly 100 percent pure olive oil.

Ideally, the bottle identifies where the olives come from, as well as the date harvested (you want oil harvested within two years).

Understanding Carbohydrates and Blood Glucose

Chocolate, cake, pizza, rice, beans, honey, broccoli, carrots, arugula . . . these are all carbohydrates. Carbohydrates are made up of monosaccharides (simple sugars), although the complexity and type of carbohydrates vary. For example, honey consists of monosaccharides (simple sugars, the simplest form of carbohydrates), where rice and beans are made up of polysaccharides, which are long chains of mono-saccharides, making them complex carbohydrates. When we eat foods containing digestible carbohydrates, most are broken down into glucose during digestion and metabolism, though some may be converted to other simple sugars like fructose. But not all carbohydrates are digested in the same way or at the same rate. So they affect our blood glucose levels differently.

Balanced blood glucose is one of the key elements to achieving long-lasting health.

Keeping blood glucose levels stable is crucial for reducing inflammation and lowering the risk of disease. More balanced blood glucose means better energy and a healthier body. A spike in glucose is a rapid increase in blood sugar followed by a rapid drop, known as *hypoglycemia*. This drop makes you reach for another snack because your energy crashes. This happens when we eat ultraprocessed simple carbohydrates like cakes, pizza, or even fruits very high in sugar.

Frequent spikes and drops in glucose levels can make you tired and damage every tissue, organ, and artery in your body. The more processed and simple carbohydrates you consume, the more your glucose spikes, leading to faster aging and a higher likelihood of disease. Simple carbohydrates include sugars that end in "ose," such as sucrose (table sugar), fructose (fruit sugar), and lactose (milk sugar).

This is where choosing complex carbohydrates like broccoli, onions, and leafy greens are the best for living well. These complex carbohydrates have lots of fiber and nutrients, which means they don't cause glucose spikes and drops. They keep you balanced and energized.

Health Tip:
Monitor Your Glucose and Insulin Levels

1. *Check fasting insulin.* Ask your doctor to check your fasting insulin annually. Increased insulin levels are a more sensitive marker of metabolic disease than fasting glucose levels.

2. *Use a continuous glucose monitor (CGM).* A CGM helps you see how different foods, stress levels, and meal timings affect your blood sugar levels 24-7. This allows you to make informed choices immediately. A CGM is a wearable device that tracks your blood glucose level in real time, for about two weeks. It gives you a clear picture on how your body responds to food, stress, sleep, and exercise so you can better understand your body

> and make lifestyle choices that serve your health. There are multiple models on the market. I have tried a couple and have been wearing the Levels CGM ever since the company started, and I love it.

Why Glucose Matters

Glucose is essential for energy, from your brain to your muscles, but it's toxic in high amounts. It damages your dream team. Research states that healthy blood glucose levels range from 70 to 100 milligrams per deciliter, but I like to see it closer to 70 to 80. An 80 milligram per deciliter glucose level means there's less than one teaspoon of glucose—about 4 grams of sugar—in your entire bloodstream. Imagine that! However, the average American consumes about thirty teaspoons of sugar a day from grains, starches, and sweets.

By reducing your sugar intake, you can reduce inflammation, keep your mitochondria and microbiome healthy, and ensure your hormones are produced in balanced amounts. Ultimately, you'll feel, function, and look better.

The Danger of Insulin Resistance

If you keep eating simple, processed carbohydrates daily, your pancreas will produce more and more insulin to respond to the glucose coming in. And for this process to work, the receptors on the cells have to respond to the insulin so the glucose can be taken up by the liver, muscle, or fat cells, and be used for making energy in the mitochondria.

At some point, though, if you are not burning the glucose by moving your body and you are overloading your system, the receptors get tired, which is called *insulin resistance*. This is the hallmark of most chronic diseases such as diabetes, heart disease, hypertension, and obesity.

Insulin resistance is like wearing earplugs while someone is shouting at you—you cannot hear them. The insulin has nowhere to go, and it remains high in the blood, causing inflammation that leads to many issues if not addressed. Without question, insulin resistance is the most common health problem, and it increases the risk of every single disease.[34]

The good news is, once you eliminate processed simple carbohydrates (baked goods, breads, sugary drinks, and the like), your body will stop craving them and you will heal. Trust me. I was the person back in Slovakia who could eat two bars of Milka chocolate a day. Those were the days!

A Few Tips to Stop Sugar Cravings

1. Use 1 tablespoon of apple cider vinegar (acetic acid) for every meal/every dressing or put it in 8 ounces of water and drink that.
2. Start each meal with fiber and protein to fill yourself up and decrease your cravings.
3. Try drinking water with a little bit of salt.

Be Sure to Get Your Fiber

Fiber is a complex carbohydrate that is essential for gut health; it acts as the primary food source for your beneficial gut bacteria. Just as we need oxygen to live, bacteria need fiber to live. If you don't feed the microbes, they will start eating you, literally. They'll start munching on the lining in your gut, the barrier that protects you. Imagine having holes in your lining. That's called *leaky gut*, which can also lead to a condition called *leaky brain*. This is unfortunately a very common problem, and it leads to harmful substances like toxins, microbes, and undigested food particles leaking into the bloodstream, triggering inflammation and immune responses.

Your body doesn't fully break down fiber. That's because humans lack the enzymes to digest most types of fiber found in plant foods. Instead, fiber travels through your small intestine and feeds those amazing gut buddies in the colon who work their magic to keep you feeling, functioning, and looking amazing.

Beneficial bacteria ferment fiber, producing postbiotics that are vital compounds for our health. So be sure to put enough fiber-rich plants on your plate. The USDA's Dietary Guidelines for Americans recommends daily fiber intake of twenty-five grams for women and thirty-one grams for men, yet the average American adult consumes only sixteen grams.[35] We used to eat one hundred grams of fiber a day![36] I aim to get fifty grams a day and recommend you, too, aim for this amount to keep your colon, gut, brain, and every other organ healthy.

Types of Fiber

The world of fiber can be complex, but to keep things simple, we'll focus on two main categories: **soluble** and **insoluble** fiber.

Soluble Fiber

Soluble fiber absorbs water, forming a gel-like substance in your gut. It helps lower glucose levels and cholesterol while also feeding the beneficial bacteria in your gut. These bacteria ferment soluble fiber, producing short-chain fatty acids like butyrate, which supports heart, brain, and immune health by reducing inflammation and promoting cellular function.

A specific type of soluble fiber, prebiotic fiber, feeds your gut bacteria. Resistant starch, a type of prebiotic fiber, resists digestion and nourishes gut bacteria. Prebiotics are found in foods like onions, garlic, leeks, asparagus, bananas, Jerusalem artichokes, dandelion greens, and chicory root. Resistant starch can also be found in unripe bananas, cooked-and-cooled potatoes, and rice.

Examples of soluble fiber include:

- Pectins: Found in legumes, oranges, apples, and pears
- Psyllium husk: A fiber supplement often used to improve digestion
- Acacia fiber: Gentle on the stomach and easily added to smoothies or water
- Flax seeds: Rich in mucilage, a soluble fiber that supports heart health
- Beta-glucans: Found in mushrooms like turkey tail, lion's mane, and reishi
- Other sources: Beans, vegetables, fruits, Jerusalem artichokes, and chicory root (rich in inulin)

Insoluble Fiber

Insoluble fiber acts like a natural broom for your digestive system. It does not dissolve in water and helps add bulk to your stool, speeding up the movement of food through the

stomach and intestines. This supports regular bowel movements, helps prevent constipation, and aids detoxification.
But it may irritate people with sensitive digestive systems,
such as those with irritable bowel syndrome (IBS).

Examples of foods high in insoluble fiber include:
- Whole grains: Wheat bran, brown rice
- Vegetables: Cauliflower, green beans, potatoes
  with skin
- Nuts and seeds: Almonds, walnuts, flaxseeds,
  sunflower seeds
- Fruits: Apples with skin, berries, pears with skin
- Legumes: Kidney beans, lentils, chickpeas

Some supplements with primarily insoluble fiber include:
- Wheat bran
- Psyllium husk (contains both soluble and insol-
  uble fiber)
- Methylcellulose

Most plants contain both soluble and insoluble fiber,
though in varying proportions. While it's generally best to get
fiber from whole foods, supplements can be helpful for those
struggling to meet their fiber needs through food alone.

When our incredible gut buddies chew on fiber, they
create metabolic byproducts of fermented fibers known as
postbiotics, which include compounds like short-chain fatty
acids (SCFAs)—acetate, propionate, and butyrate. These
SCFAs are critical in reducing risks associated with diabetes,
obesity, and heart disease. Butyrate, for instance, helps
reduce inflammation and is being studied for its potential
protective effects against colon cancer.[37]

Did you know that 70 percent of your immune system is made in the gut?[38] That's right. Ninety percent of serotonin (the happy hormone) is made in the gut, as is about 50 percent of your dopamine.[39] A healthier gut simply means a healthier and happier you. Remember, hormones regulate your mood.

The benefits of fiber extend further. Fiber slows digestion and manages blood sugar levels. High-fiber foods are also more filling, which can help you control your appetite and maintain a healthy body weight.

Whole grains are a good fiber source, but it's essential to consume them in their whole and unprocessed form to retain their nutritional benefits. Processed grains, like those found in white bread or pasta, have had their fiber and nutrients significantly reduced or completely removed, leading to a flood of glucose in the blood, which results in blood sugar spikes and crashes. There is no more fiber to feed your gut buddies.

Hidden Troublemakers to Avoid

Wheat is a grain that I suggest most of us avoid eating, as it has been extremely modified through breeding. Gluten's main proteins, gliadins, increase zonulin production in the gut. We need some zonulin, which is important for regulating the tight junctions in our gut lining. But too much zonulin, as mentioned in the previous chapter on toxins, causes the loosening of tight junctions between intestinal cells, allowing toxins to pass through into our bloodstream, which alerts the immune system to attack and creates inflammation.

Corn consumption should also be limited. Ninety percent of corn grown in the US is genetically modified,[40] producing toxins that poke holes in the cells of the intestine that, again, lead to inflammation.

Tips to Increase Your Daily Fiber

- Steam and cool your potatoes before you eat them. This reduced heat makes them less glycemic. Cooling transforms the starch to a more resistant starch. When you bake potatoes, the molecules expand, making the food more glycemic.
- Add a handful of beans and legumes to your daily meals.
- Add leeks, onions, garlic to your daily meals.
- Make a batch of vegetable soup every week.
- Bake vegetables on low heat.
- Add fermented vegetables to every meal, which are also rich in probiotics—healthy bacteria for your gut (unless you have histamine intolerance, in which case I do not recommend any fermented foods).
- Prepare three bowls of vegetables for every day, ready to eat.
- Have cleaned and cut carrots, bell peppers, and celery ready to munch on throughout the day.
- Enjoy blueberries and apples when they are in season.
- Focus on quality and variety. Switch up your plant foods. If you routinely eat the same vegetables, try something new. Enjoy experiencing different flavors and textures. Most importantly, have fun with your food! You'll grow more diverse "friends" in your gut, which is the ultimate goal.

Fermented Foods

Fermentation acts as a natural preservative, extending the shelf life of foods by producing beneficial bacteria and acids that inhibit the growth of harmful pathogens. Fermented foods have numerous health benefits, supporting everything from digestion and immunity to mental health and weight management.

Fermented foods contain probiotics, which are beneficial bacteria that help balance the gut microbiome and improve digestion. As we already learned, we need a good amount of different, healthy gut buddies to live well.

Examples of fermented foods:

- Plain kefir
- Plain yogurt
- Sauerkraut
- Kimchi
- Miso
- Raw apple cider vinegar, unfiltered
- Aged cheeses
- Cocoa powder

A Stanford study found that daily intake of fermented foods increases the diversity of gut buddies.[41] The more different types of microbes present in your gut, the better you feel, function, and look.

Make fermented foods part of your daily meals. But be careful if you have a genetic predisposition to histamine intolerance.[42] Fermented foods contain bacteria that produce large amounts of histamine. Many people do not know they struggle with this histamine intolerance. One way to find out is to do a comprehensive genetic testing and look for these genes and their function: diamine oxidase (DAO), histamine N-methyltransferase (HNMT), monoamine oxidase (MAO), and amiloride-binding protein1 (ABP1). Great resources for genetic testing and understanding genes is Dr. Ben Lynch's book *Dirty Genes: A Breakthrough Program to Treat the Root Cause of Illness and Optimize Your Health.*

Histamine is important as it supports our ability to focus, think, learn, and stay awake. Histamine also supports our immune system, allowing it to respond when needed for healing cuts or scrapes. When we have too much histamine, however, it causes inflammation and many other health issues.

Remember that a significant percent of your immune processes and your overall health are linked to your microbiome, so feed those good bugs lots of plant and fermented real foods.[43]

Take a Moment

All right, that was a lot to take in, I know! I've distilled the most essential information to help you feel more empowered. Take a moment to breathe, write down any notes or thoughts, and prepare yourself for the next exciting part—learning about my absolute favorite plant.

I Love Sprouts—And I Hope You Will Too

Sprouts are a great source of minerals, vitamins, and phytochemicals. Some varieties, like pea sprouts, are also high in amino acids. These are true superheroes in removing toxins. Buy them, grow them, eat them.

Broccoli sprouts in particular have up to one hundred times more glucoraphanin than mature broccoli.[44] Glucoraphanin is a nutrient that gets converted into a powerful health-boosting molecule called sulforaphane by an enzyme called myrosinase. This enzyme gets activated when you crush, chop, or chew the broccoli sprouts but becomes inactive if you cook them for too long or at high temperatures.

What we really want is the sulforaphane, the active molecule, because it has amazing benefits. Sulforaphane helps protect your brain and can reduce the risk of cancer.

Sulforaphane lowers DNA damage by lowering oxidative stress and inflammation, which are central to cancer, aging, neurodegenerative diseases, and other ailments. Sulforaphane removes benzene from the lungs, heals your intestine lining, and kills weak cells that would otherwise cause trouble. Benzene is a harmful chemical that is found in the air due to industrial emissions, vehicle exhaust, and cigarette smoke. It is a known carcinogen.

To increase the amount of sulforaphane you get from sprouts, you can freeze fresh sprouts, which can increase the concentration by up to two times.[45]

How to Enjoy Sprouts Every Day
- Use them in your pesto.
- Blend a handful of sprouts into pasta sauce.
- Blend sprouts into smoothies.
- Mix them into your salads.
- Be creative—add them to everything!

A study published in the journal *Cancer Epidemiology, Biomarkers and Prevention* shows the power of eating cruciferous vegetables, like broccoli sprouts. People with bladder cancer who ate only four servings of raw broccoli per month had a 57 percent reduction in bladder cancer mortality, and a 43 percent reduction in all-cause mortality (this is compared to those who just had one serving per month). A case-control study found that a higher intake of cruciferous vegetables was associated with a 40 percent lower odds of pancreatic cancer.[46]

What a powerful plant, right? I hope I have convinced you to add sprouts to your daily meal planning.

Herbs and Spices Provide a Lot More than Flavor

Each sprinkle of paprika, oregano, garlic, cumin, coriander, and rosemary (and your other favorite herbs and spices) not only adds depth and aroma to your dishes, but it also brings a host of health benefits. In fact, herbs and spices are some of the most nutrient- and antioxidant-dense foods on the planet. Some have antimicrobial properties, meaning they can help kill or stop the growth of harmful bacteria, and others have antifungal effects, helping kill or stop the growth of fungi, which can cause infections. Many spices also rank higher in antioxidant activity than fruits and vegetables.[47]

Tips for Herbs and Spices

- Always buy organic herbs and spices in glass jars. Keep them in a dark, cool place.
- Notice the expiration date on the jars, as herbs and spices are very sensitive to oxidation.
- Don't put your fingers in the jar, as this can infect the contents with bacteria.
- I prefer to buy my herbs and spices directly from the supplier to avoid oxidation from them sitting on store shelves for months. My favorites are Mountain Rose Herbs and Organic Spices Inc.

Micronutrients: The Tiny Powerhouses of Health

Despite their small size, these essential nutrients play a crucial role in maintaining your health and well-being. So, what exactly are micronutrients? They include vitamins and minerals found in all real, whole foods. The term *vitamin* shares a root with the word *vital*, underscoring their importance for health.

Vitamins are generally divided into two categories: fat-soluble and water-soluble.

Fat-Soluble Vitamins

- Vitamin A: Think of this as the headlights for your car, crucial for vision, immune function, and skin health.
- Vitamin D: Imagine it as the sturdy foundation of a house, essential for bone health, immune health, and calcium in bone absorption. Vitamin D is also classified as a hormone.
- Vitamin E: This antioxidant acts like the body's natural shield, protecting cells from damage.
- Vitamin K: Necessary for blood clotting and bone health, Vitamin K2 directs calcium from the arteries to the bones, ensuring it goes where it's needed. Pairing Vitamin D3 with K2 is like having a GPS for calcium, guiding it properly to support overall bone health.

Here are some foods where you can get each of these vitamins:

- Vitamin A: beef liver, sweet potatoes, carrots
- Vitamin D: fatty fish, cod liver oil
- Vitamin E: sunflower seeds, almonds, spinach
- Vitamin K: brussels sprouts, kale, spinach

- Vitamin C: acerola cherries, red bell peppers, kiwi
- Vitamin B
  - B1: sunflower seeds, macadamia nuts
  - B2: beef liver, yogurt
  - B3: chicken, turkey
  - B5: avocados, sunflower seeds, mushrooms
  - B6: chickpeas, turkey, pistachios
  - B7: egg yolks, nuts, sweet potatoes
  - B9: lentils, asparagus
  - B12: beef liver, sardines, clams

Water-Soluble Vitamins

- Vitamin C: This is your body's superhero, boosting the immune system, enhancing skin health, and providing antioxidant protection.
- B Vitamins: These are your body's mechanics, influencing mood, hormone regulation, energy levels, detoxification, and memory. They are essential for converting food into cellular energy, acting as copilots for enzymes in various biochemical functions. They are absolutely essential in order to lower oxidative stress, and for proper digestion, brain health, and increased energy. If you have genetic variations, you have an even higher need for B vitamins. Amino acids and B vitamins work closely together in the body, each playing a critical role in building and maintaining health. Amino acids are the building blocks for enzymes, which are essential for various bodily functions. B vitamins, on the other hand, activate and support these enzymes, enabling them to perform their tasks effectively. Amino acids make enzymes, and B vitamins make the enzymes work.

Do you see how important it is to have a variety of real, whole foods? We can't isolate and separate. There is this incredible teamwork happening inside our bodies. It's so beautiful when you envision all these workers helping each other, working together making you feel and function your best.

Minerals are another essential part of this micronutrient team, and they're divided into two categories based on the amounts needed.

Macrominerals (Needed in Larger Amounts)

- Calcium: Think of it as the building block for bones and muscles.
- Phosphorus: Working alongside calcium, it is vital for bone health and energy production.
- Magnesium: This multitasker is involved in more than three hundred biochemical reactions, including muscle and nerve function, sleep regulation, thyroid health, antioxidant glutathione production, DNA repair, and energy production.[48] Imagine it as the repair crew for your DNA, preventing damage and activating vitamin C for more effectiveness. Green plants are rich in magnesium, so as your mother told you, eat your greens—and plenty of them! (Note: Athletes and those who sweat daily need more magnesium, as it is lost through sweat.)
- Sodium: Essential for fluid balance and nerve function, like the electrolyte that keeps your body's battery charged.
- Potassium: Vital for heart function, muscle contraction, as well as cell hydration.

- Chloride: Important for fluid balance and digestion.
- Sulfur: A component of certain amino acids and vitamins, like the structural support beams in a building.

Trace Minerals (Needed in Smaller Amounts)

- Iron: Necessary for oxygen transport in the blood, like the delivery truck for your cells.
- Zinc: Important for immune function, wound healing, and DNA synthesis.
- Copper: Involved in iron metabolism and enzyme function, acting like the assistant manager in nutrient processing.
- Manganese: Supports bone formation, metabolism, and cell hydration.
- Iodine: Essential for thyroid hormone production, like the thermostat regulating your body's energy.
- Selenium: Acts as an antioxidant and supports thyroid function.
- Chromium: Involved in macronutrient metabolism.
- Molybdenum: Supports enzyme function.

Eating a variety of real, whole foods ensures you get all the micronutrients needed to live well. Just as a diverse array of tools is needed to fix different problems in a house, a varied diet provides all the nutrients your body needs to function optimally.

Here are some examples of where to find each of these micronutrients:

- Calcium: dairy, sardines with bones, tofu
- Phosphorus: chicken, dairy products, pumpkin seeds
- Magnesium: pumpkin seeds, avocados, black beans

- Sodium: seaweed, celery, beetroot
- Potassium: avocados, bananas, white beans
- Chloride: table salt, tomatoes
- Sulfur: garlic, onions, eggs
- Iron: red meat, lentils, dark chocolate
- Zinc: oysters, beef, pumpkin seeds
- Selenium: Brazil nuts, eggs
- Copper: beef liver, oysters, dark chocolate
- Manganese: pineapple, nuts (hazelnuts, pecans), brown rice
- Iodine: seaweed, fish
- Chromium: broccoli, whole grains
- Molybdenum: legumes, nuts, whole grains

Let's Take Another Small Break for a Moment

This chapter has covered a lot of information about food, and I'm sure you are connecting the dots now, understanding that everything we choose to put into our mouths has a direct and specific effect on our mood, behavior, and overall health—through mitochondria and gut bacteria functions.

It takes time to incorporate this knowledge into your lifestyle. In that spirit, here are some simple reminders when thinking about food:

Buy Quality Food

Choose products with these labels, depending on the food ingredient: wild, pasture-raised, organic, raw, sprouted.

Connect to Your Body

Notice how your body responds when eating a certain food—in the moment, right now. Do you feel good? Keep eating it.

Bloated? Tired? Heart racing? Feeling irritated? Skin itchy? Stop eating it. Listen to your body—it's always right. A food that is healthy for one person can create a problem in another person.

Enjoy Variety

Experiment with different plants, sprouts, meats, and fish. Even if you are eating healthy foods, the microbiome needs a diversity of fibers for bacteria diversity. You can keep it simple and diverse at the same time.

Other Areas of Food that Affect Our Health

When to Eat

The timing of your meals can significantly impact how you feel and function.

Your body runs on an internal twenty-four-hour cycle called the *circadian rhythm*. This assures that hormones, hunger cues, bowel movements, energy levels, sleepiness, and all other body functions work on schedule. When we follow the circadian rhythm, we power through days effortlessly and sleep beautifully. Our bodies love routine and predictability. Following our natural biological clock and eating on a somewhat regular schedule leads to better digestion, increased detoxification, improved brain health, and overall feeling and functioning great.

Just like the Earth rotates around the sun, you can't escape the circadian rhythm, and can't change or influence it. If we do not follow nature's powerful cycle, we end up feeling miserable.

The good news is that repairing our twenty-four-hour cycle takes changing just a few key habits related to meal timing. Once back on track, everything effortlessly clicks, and we regain that vibrant flow state automatically!

When the sun goes down, it's time for rest. Our suprachiasmatic nucleus (SCN), the part of our brain that regulates our circadian rhythm, tells the pineal gland to start releasing melatonin to get our bodies ready for sleep. Almost every cell in the body has melatonin receptors. When melatonin is released at night, it binds to receptors on the pancreas.

This gives the pancreas the message, "Hey, it's nighttime. It's time to take a break and repair." That means insulin secretion from the pancreas is inhibited; it goes down, which means our cells aren't great at breaking down food at night. This is why the whole digestive system is designed to metabolize food best earlier in the day.

The movement of stool through our gut and the production of saliva, stomach acid, and digestive enzymes all go down significantly when melatonin is being released and while we're asleep.

We are not supposed to eat at any time, or all the time!

This is why it is a good idea to avoid eating after the sun goes down, or to eat lighter meals like plants and fish. There are circadian rhythms in insulin secretion and glucose metabolism that can affect how the body responds to food at different times of day. Consuming food, especially simple carbohydrates and sugars, close to bedtime leads to insulin release, which can inhibit growth hormone secretion. GH is crucial for muscle repair and overall body healing during deep sleep.

Tips for Healthy Meal Timing

Eat high-carbohydrate meals earlier.

If you are going to eat highly processed carbohydrates, aim to eat them at lunch rather than at dinner when your digestive enzymes are their peak levels. Another great tip is to fill up on protein, fats, and fiber first to slow down the flood of glucose from pizza or cake. For example, when I want to have some popcorn and watch a movie, I plan it in the early afternoon, and I eat a large bowl of arugula and avocado salad with pumpkin seeds and hemp seeds first. (This is my favorite salad.)

Adopt a time-restricted eating window.

Finish eating at least three to four hours before bedtime to allow for most of your food to digest.

Follow a consistent eating schedule.

Eating at the same or close to the same times each day is easier on your digestion due to the circadian rhythm.

Sometimes, it's good to not to eat at all.

From time to time, the body needs a break from all the work involved in digestion, as it takes a significant amount of energy and resources. The no-eating time window is crucial to give the body time to repair. The body can't repair well if it's constantly digesting food, breaking it down and building new molecules.

This concept of not eating, known as *fasting* or *time-restricted eating*, has become popular in modern society. There is no strict definition for *fasting*. Actually, we fast naturally while we're sleeping. Whenever we don't consume any calories, we are fasting.

If you are constantly eating from 6:00 a.m. to 10:00 p.m., and add snacks on top of eating three complete meals, that is a constant stress on your body. Your body has to be producing digestive enzymes for too many hours, and your immune system is exhausted from overworking. Just like you have breaks from work, your body needs a break from food. It's important to eat within a time-restricted window, which allows the body time to rest. During rest, your organs have time to do some cleanup. It's hard to do a deep cleaning of your kitchen if someone is constantly cooking and using the space.

Consider that it takes approximately five hours for food to fully digest, depending on the food. Heavier, fatty meals take longer to digest. So, if you finish dinner at 8:00 p.m., you are still digesting at midnight. Having late-night food once in a while, if you are healthy overall, is not a problem; your body can handle it. But constant late-night eating throws our natural clocks out of sync, causing health problems.

When it comes to fasting or TRE (time-restricted eating), I suggest you choose what method works best for your health goals. I also recommend talking to a functional medicine practitioner if you have any serious health issues and are considering fasting longer than twenty-four hours or more.

Metabolic Health

Fasting helps improve metabolic flexibility, allowing your body to easily switch between burning carbohydrates (sugar) and fat for energy. When you are metabolically healthy, your body can create energy from stored fat, glycogen in your muscles, and ketones from the liver. When we overeat carbs and eat every two hours, we are not metabolically flexible or healthy. Fasting is like practicing switching between burning available carbohydrates (when you eat) and burning fat for energy (when you're not eating). This switch enhances your energy levels. Conversely, constant eating keeps your body reliant on glucose, making it less efficient at burning fat and more metabolically inflexible. This inflexibility can lead to feeling sluggish and eventually developing metabolic diseases like obesity and type 2 diabetes.

Other health benefits of fasting are:

- **Autophagy.** Fasting triggers autophagy, where your body removes damaged cells and recycles parts for repairs.[49]
- **Mitophagy.** This clears out dysfunctional mitochondria.[50]
- **Cancer prevention.** By depriving cancer cells of fuel, fasting can help in cleaning up sick and uncontrolled cells.[51]
- **Production of brain-derived neurotrophic factor (BDNF).** Fasts can increase BDNF levels, promoting better brain function and cognitive health. BDNF is the protein you want a lot of for a healthy brain. It works like a soil fertilizer for your brain. Another great benefit of high BDNFs is that as it goes up, leptin, the hunger hormone, goes down. Similarly, high-intensity interval training (HIIT), as will be discussed in the chapter on movement, also boosts BDNF.[52]

Implementing Time-Restricted Eating (TRE)

Adopting a time-restricted eating (TRE) window means having specific periods for eating and not eating. For example, a 16:8 pattern means you fast for sixteen hours and consume food only during the remaining eight hours of the day. Evidence suggests that TRE improves cognitive function, supports weight loss, and reduces systemic inflammation.[53] This downtime allows the body to focus on DNA and cellular repair and restoration rather than digestion. DNA repair is crucial because it maintains the integrity of our genetic information, preventing mutations that can lead to diseases like cancer and promoting overall cellular health. By allowing time for DNA repair, TRE helps ensure long-term health and vitality.

I practice 16:8 or 18:6 time-restricted eating daily, which means eating in a six-to-eight-hour window and not eating for sixteen to eighteen hours. Sometimes I do a twenty-four-hour fast, paying close attention to my menstrual cycle, sleep, and exercise plans.

If you are new to TRE and fasting, start with shorter fasts or TRE and gradually increase the duration to allow your body to adapt. Restrict eating for twelve to fourteen hours overnight and try to grow into the habit of fourteen to sixteen hours of no eating.[54]

What Happens During a Prolonged Fast

Understand that prolonged fasting is a type of stress known as hormesis. This kind of stress is important because it triggers the body's adaptive responses, making you stronger and more resilient. It helps to improve cellular function, enhance metabolism, and promote overall health. By challenging the body in manageable ways, such as through fasting, we can stimulate positive changes and improve our ability to handle future stresses.

Sometimes fasting can be too stressful for some of us. Extended fasting can raise levels of cortisol, a stress hormone that regulates metabolism. This may trigger the production of glucose from noncarbohydrate sources, like muscle proteins, but short-term fasting usually doesn't lead to major muscle loss in healthy individuals.

While fasting lowers insulin, the balance between cortisol, glucose, and insulin varies from person to person. Prolonged hormone elevation could contribute to inflammation and metabolic stress.

If you're used to frequent meals, especially ones high in carbs, your body may struggle to switch to burning fat for energy, reducing its metabolic flexibility and making fasting harder to adapt to.

Fasting affects everyone differently. That's why I believe it's a good idea to start slow, pay attention to how you feel, and do a deeper dive into how to fast properly.

Hydration during any long TRE and fast is extremely important because your body will be burning fat, and fat stores toxins. You don't want to recycle toxins in your body that are being released during a fast. You need to get them out through sweat, urine, stool, and breath.

Entering and Breaking a Fast

You may be asking what breaks a fast. Even lemon juice has calories, so a true fast is nothing but water, herbal teas, or pure coffee. You are breaking your fast with your first caloric meal or drink.

Make sure the last meal before your fast, and the first meal after your fast, are low in simple carbohydrates and higher in fat, fiber, and protein. This ensures you will have a low glycemic response and an easier way of switching to fat burning. Otherwise, you'll feel miserable, which will make it difficult to fast; as your glucose spikes and drops, you may become hypoglycemic, which means you'll become hungry.

As for how to break the fast, I suggest starting slow and not overloading your system with calories. I like to start with a vegetable or organic bone broth to prepare my digestion for solid food coming in. Then I eat some clean protein, like salmon or sardines, to replenish the loss, along with steamed or lightly sautéed vegetables. After a fast the body has a harder time digesting, because it was on a nice break of making digestive enzymes. Your microbiome has also been changed during this time. If you load your body with a large serving of raw vegetables, you may get bloated.

Pay Attention to How You Eat

Imagine trying to enjoy a fine meal while running a race; it just doesn't work well. If you aren't breathing calmly, sitting down, and savoring each meal with all your senses, your body won't produce the right amount of digestive enzymes needed to break down food. This can lead to nutrient deficiencies and inflammation because your microbiome cannot thrive in a stressed environment. As I mentioned earlier, it's not just about what you eat but what you digest. Effective digestion only happens when you are relaxed.

Digestion starts in your mouth with digestive enzymes produced in saliva. These enzymes are released when we are in a calm, parasympathetic state. As you chew, you signal your stomach to increase acid production, preparing it to break down the food. Eating in rushed or stressful ways leads to imbalances in digestion and assimilation due to low enzyme production. Food then moves into the intestines before it's adequately broken down.

You must fully chew to digest your food and get all the benefits from it. So, take the time to sit down, breathe calmly, and enjoy your meals. Think of it as giving your body the pit stop it needs to refuel effectively.

Mindful Eating Tips for Health

When my family and I sit down to eat, we pause, take a breath, smell the food, and say thank-you for the food we are about to consume. That process takes one minute at the most. In just sixty seconds we completely change the course of the meal, all for the better.

Do this with each meal:

1. Put away distractions (phones, books, TV, etc.).
2. Sit down.
3. Take a moment to look at and smell the food.
4. Take a deep breath and express gratitude for the meal.
5. Chew mindfully to aid digestion.

Be Careful How Much You Eat

Overeating beyond your nutritional requirements can cause a number of problems. For one, you will gain weight and have a higher risk for associated diseases like diabetes. Overeating also causes your pancreas to work much harder, which eventually leads to digestive discomfort due to constant stress. [55]

The Order of Foods

The order in which you eat your food matters if you eat processed carbohydrates and sugary foods and want to keep your glucose levels balanced. I suggest always eating plants first to feed your gut microbiome. This nourishes your gut buddies, and it allows for slower digestion, which helps prevent glucose spikes if you are having bread, pizza, or pasta. Next, have high-quality, clean protein to support your brain, immune system, and muscles.

For example, if you want to enjoy bread or pasta, start with a bowl of broccoli with a drizzle of olive oil and herbs. Then, have some salmon or bison before the pasta or bread. You'll eat less pasta, still enjoy it, get your favorite processed carbs in, and avoid glucose spikes, which means no inflammation in your arteries!

How to Prepare Your Food

We now understand what to eat, when to eat it, how to eat for the best possible digestion, and how we should eat foods in a certain order for better health. But we can't forget about the importance of how we prepare our food. How we cook our food affects not only its taste, but also its nutritional value.

Cooking foods at a high enough temperature to sear and crisp them may produce tasty results for some. But it turns out that food that becomes dark brown or black during the cooking process is packed with compounds like acrylamides and advanced glycation end products (AGEs).[56] Remember these from the chapter on toxins? They are pro-oxidant, proinflammatory, and damaging to cells in the brain and DNA.

AGEs in particular are dangerous because they can damage brain cells, leading to diseases like Alzheimer's.[57] They do this by messing with proteins called *tau proteins* that help transport nutrients in brain cells, causing blockages and cell death, which contribute to memory loss and cognitive decline.

In people with diabetes, high blood sugar can increase the production of AGEs, further damaging cells and promoting complications like heart disease and even cancer.[58] AGEs are also found in ultraprocessed factory foods, which is one more reason to avoid them.

As you can see, these are toxic molecules. They create reactive oxygen species (ROS) and cause cell death, organ damage, and mitochondrial dysfunction.

AGEs are so unhealthy, in fact, that many functional medicine doctors are now starting to look at AGE levels as a marker of overall health.

How to Limit the Production of AGEs

Balance your blood sugar. AGEs tend to accumulate more in people with elevated blood sugar levels; eliminate or keep sugar and alcohol to a real minimum, depending on your overall health goals.

Eat spices and plants. These are natural antioxidants. Vitamin C, curcumin, and quercetin from plants hinder AGE production in the body. The polyphenols in olive leaf have shown success in liming formation of AGEs. Use a lot of spices like rosemary, turmeric, oregano, and garlic on your food.

Use low temperatures for cooking. Use a slow, low-temperature, high-moisture pressure cooker for healthier cooking. Pressure cooking at lower temperatures can retain about 90 to 95 percent of food nutrients, outperforming methods like steaming, roasting, and boiling.[59]

Marinate food in acidic marinades like lemon juice. This can reduce production of AGEs by 50 percent.[60]

Cook with a bit of water. Continually adding water to retain moisture is a great way to eat for feeling and functioning well.

"This All Sounds Great, but I Love Eating Out"

We all love the experience of dining out: the ambiance, service, delicious food, and not having to cook or do the dishes. However, dining out can expose you to a plate full of toxins. If you dine out regularly, you might start to connect the dots between your meals and feeling tired all the time, having headaches, joint pain, and weight gain, or struggling with bloating.

Helpful Tips for Healthier Dining Out

- *Plan ahead.* Look at the menu online and choose your meal before going to the restaurant.
- *Skip the bread.* Say no to the bread basket.
- *Simplify your salad.* Avoid salad dressings, croutons, and candied nuts. Instead, ask for lemon and olive oil.
- *Avoid charred and fried food.* Ask for your food to be steamed, sautéed, or grilled without black marks.
- *Choose vegetables wisely.* Ask for your vegetables to be steamed or sautéed with butter. In fact, start your meal

this way. You can order side dishes like brussels sprouts or broccoli instead of salads.

I understand that making special requests at restaurants can feel daunting, but always remember why you're on this journey of health and healing. Ask the waitstaff with kindness and confidence. Most restaurants are accommodating, and I always tip well in return when they are understanding.

Eat for Yourself, Not for Others

Many of my clients tell me, "I want to eat healthier, but my friends don't. They tease me or dismiss my health goals, making it hard to enjoy our time together." It's heartbreaking to see some of my clients prioritizing fitting in over their own well-being, even though they truly want to improve their health. Choosing between relationships and health shouldn't be this hard, but it often is. It takes patience, support, and a lot of strategizing to move from feeling stuck to confidently standing up for your health needs. Together, we work on building that confidence—because everyone deserves to feel their best while enjoying the company of others.

When you think about it, it's odd that we feel like we have to justify wanting to improve our health. How backward!

Share Your Goals, Own Your Plate!

Don't try to change the attitudes of your family members or friends. Here is where open and honest communication, without stories and assumptions, is important.

Explain, don't defend! Tell people how you feel and why you have specific lifestyle goals. Tell them that their support is meaningful to you. Make food compromises that work for both parties if this is what you want, such as planning meals together that include options for everyone's preferences. When you are open and honest about your own needs, the rest is up to them. True friends and loving family members will support you and cheer you on even if they do not eat the way you do.

Lead by example and demonstrate the benefits of healthy eating through your own actions. So many times, hearing about and seeing positive changes in someone else will inspire others to make similar changes themselves. Everyone wants to feel amazing, and once they see you change, they may want to follow. And if not, that's their choice as well.

In many cases, spouses and partners are not on the same health page. This is where personal coaching is a good approach for finding mutual agreement and understanding.

Of course, changing yourself is hard enough; it's even more challenging (maybe impossible) to change others. Take pride in your decision to make a better and healthier life for yourself. Think about creating a support network outside of your circle. Join online communities, find a workout buddy, or participate in group coaching sessions where you can connect with like-minded individuals. You don't have to be alone in this transformation. Surround yourself with people who are on the same path as you: the path to optimal, joyful living.

Set boundaries around your own health habits and make it clear that you are not willing to compromise. Designate certain areas of the kitchen for healthy foods only, and schedule regular exercise time without interruption.

I share all of this based on personal experience. None of my friends eat the way I eat; neither does my husband. For years, I have been bringing my own food on road trips, on airplanes, and to gatherings because I believe in what I am doing and I want to feel great. There is a certain confidence I exude that makes people respond with curiosity rather than admonishing me.

We become who we surround ourselves with. If your friends drink every night and have sedentary lifestyles, so will you. If people judge you, it may be beneficial to find a new circle of supportive people.

Overall, focus on your *why* and be in complete alignment with your values and beliefs. It's your life, your health—eat what's right for you, not for others.

Treat Yourself to a Treat—Once in a While

While your goal is to attain optimum health, that doesn't mean you have to make perfect choices all the time. We are humans, and it's about balance. If we are healthy we can afford to enjoy our favorite nonnutritious treats occasionally.

Here's my approach:

Choose a healthier treat option.

If you like tortilla chips like me, switch to organic, baked, low-carbohydrate crackers. Read the ingredient label to make sure you can pronounce and understand each ingredient. If you like chocolate, choose an organic, dark, fair-trade chocolate bar. Those are just a few examples. Whatever treat you have in mind, you can always find something healthier that's equally tasty as the junk variety.

Plan your treat.

Don't eat that treat anytime you feel like it. Instead, have it at the right time for your body. So have dessert for dessert, not for breakfast. Eat dessert after a lunch that ideally includes plenty of plants and protein. Eat slowly and enjoy each bite.

Enjoy, then move.

After indulging in the delicious piece of birthday cake, don't sit in front of the TV. Get out of the house and take a nice, vigorous walk.

Tip for Cravings

The more real food you eat, the fewer cravings you'll have for nonnutritious foods. Our taste receptors change; just give them a chance! The more sugar and salt you eat, the more sugar and salt you crave because you get more desensitized and the amount needs to get bigger for you to feel the same satisfaction. Of course, when you do have cravings for sweet things, be sure to follow the steps listed above—and do it seldomly.

Reading Ingredient Labels Is Nonnegotiable!

As consumers, we are responsible for our food choices. This is why we must carefully read food labels to determine what's really inside the boxes or bottles. Sadly, that's not always easy, since food labeling is designed to confuse us and complicate things.

There are so many ridiculous labels, names, and claims on the front of packaged foods attempting to convince you that you're making a healthy choice. These are empty claims only meant to catch your eye and lure you in, but they tell you nothing about the quality of the food and its ingredients. The worst part? The Food and Drug Administration (FDA) does nothing to help the consumer decipher labels and confusing misinformation.

Since the FDA won't help you, I will.

- Ignore the marketing language on the front of every packaged product.
- Always turn the packaging container over and look at the ingredients food label.
- Check the serving size. Are you going to eat the serving size amount or more?
- Look at the order of ingredients. They are always listed in descending order by weight, meaning the first ingredient is present in the highest weight, followed by the second, and so on. If the first ingredient is any kind of sugar, put it down!
- Check for added sugar. If there are more than four grams of added sugar in one serving, don't buy it.
- Check for trans fats and unrecognizable ingredients. If the label says, "partially hydrogenated," "artificial flavors," or includes ingredients you don't recognize, put it down.
- Calculate net carbohydrates. Net carbs refer to the total amount of carbohydrates in food that can significantly impact blood sugar levels! Lower net-carb foods typically have a milder effect on glucose levels. Here's how to calculate it. Start with the "total carbohydrates" listed on the nutrition label, then subtract "dietary fiber," which is the fiber we can't digest and

need for healthy gut microbiome, to determine the net carbs. The amount of net carbs you want to eat is dependent on your current health and your health goals. To give you an example, typically a low-carb diet may recommend anywhere from twenty to one hundred grams of net carbs per day for managing blood sugar levels. If your focus is on general health and well-being, net carb intake may vary from one hundred to one hundred fifty grams per day or more, depending on individual needs and activity levels. The best way to know how you respond to the net carb amounts in food is by wearing a CGM.

Teach Your Loved Ones How to Read Food Labels Too

My daughter, Summer, was four years old and already reading when her preschool teacher shared a story with a smile of admiration. She had noticed Summer would read the ingredients label before she would eat any snack a child brought into the class to share.

Interestingly, I never taught Summer to read labels. She was always in the kitchen with me, always grocery shopping with me, and she simply observed how I read food labels. This is the power we parents have. We teach by example.

Last, although it's critical to diligently read labels, most of your food should have no labels at all: fresh plants, meat, fish, nuts, and seeds.

Water: Nature's All-Purpose Remedy

Improving our health doesn't have to be complicated. Simple actions, like drinking water, can have significant benefits.

Hydration also involves water absorption inside your cells, which requires minerals, also known as electrolytes. Over two-thirds of your body's water is inside your cells. Potassium and magnesium push water into the cells through osmosis. Without adequate magnesium and potassium, water can't enter your cells effectively. Eating fresh, organic plants daily provides the minerals needed to properly hydrate your cells.

Certain drinks, like coffee, green tea, alcohol, and some fermented beverages, can dehydrate you by causing electrolyte loss. Water is the most crucial nutrient for your body, making up about 60 to 80 percent of human cells and tissues. Proper hydration supports optimal cellular functions, fine motor skills, memory, and decision-making. Inadequate water intake can lead to high blood pressure, as less water in your blood makes your heart work harder.

Remember, your immune system is most active at night. If you don't drink enough water during the day, you go to bed dehydrated, and your immune system won't function properly.

Water Tips

Avoid tap water. Most tap water contains contaminants, like disinfection byproducts or fluoride, which have a negative effect on health by disrupting your thyroid and other hormones. That said, sometimes you have no choice but to drink tap water. In those cases, filter it. Many pitcher filters can filter some disinfectant byproducts but do not trap smaller particles, notably fluoride. Check the Environmental Working Group's website, ewg.org, for good filtration system options, though to be safe, I prefer a reverse osmosis system and add minerals with real whole foods or supplements if needed; reverse osmosis removes all the junk.

Water with higher magnesium concentrations (ideally: 8.3 to 19.4 milligrams per liter) is more alkaline and, therefore, improves absorption, as I mentioned earlier. More alkaline water can reduce inflammation and blood pressure and lower the risks of cardiovascular disease, though this has nothing to do with changing the pH of your body, as some water brands suggest.

Try hydrogen-enriched water. This has a higher pH than normal tap water. One study has shown that hydrogen-enriched water reduces inflammation, likely due to improved hydration of cells.[61] You can make this type of water at home by dissolving a molecular hydrogen tablet (which contains a specific type of magnesium) in a glass of water.

Important Note: Always use glass, ceramic, or stainless-steel containers for your water. Never plastic.

How to Drink More Water

- Every night before going to bed, set out about thirty-two ounces of water.
- When you get up, go outside or open a window and drink your water while enjoying the morning light. Do this every day for the rest of your life.
- Purchase a large (at least thirty-two-ounce) stainless-steel water bottle and keep it with you throughout the day.
- Add some herbal tea to your day, and refill your bottle as needed.
- Remember, the more you sweat, the more you need to hydrate.

Respect Your Needs

Everyone has different food preferences, as well as individual reactions to specific foods. It can be challenging to develop a smart nutrition plan when you're beginning your health journey. Below are the foods that make up my lifestyle. See what works best for you!

Essentials

- Goat or sheep's milk
- Berries, apples, and seasonal fruits like nectarines and apricots
- All kinds of veggies except eggplant
- Nuts, seeds
- Nut butters
- Beans
- Sauerkraut
- Goat kefir
- Eggs
- Wild meat, wild salmon, chicken, anchovies, sardines
- Goat and sheep cheeses
- Sheep yogurt
- Wild California rice
- Herbs and seasonings
- Olive oil
- Lupini pasta
- Pasta sauce
- Tomato paste
- Cocoa powder (CocoaVia)
- Balsamic vinegar
- Apple cider vinegar

Daily Supplements
- Magnesium glycinate, malate, and L-threonate
- High-quality fish oil
- Methylated B complex
- Collagen powder and creatine
- Glutathione
- Alpha-lipoic acid
- Quercetin
- NAC and glycine
- Prebiotic fiber and probiotics
- Vitamin D3 + K2

Twelve Ways to Feel Better Every Day

1. Upon waking in the morning, drink two or more glasses of clean, filtered water.
2. Enjoy a breakfast rich in clean protein and fiber.
3. Sit down at every meal, take three breaths, look at the food, smell it, and say thank-you before you begin and chew well.
4. Eat your last meal of the day a minimum of three hours before bed. If you're a chronic late-night eater, start by moving your dinner thirty minutes earlier for one week. Be consistent.
5. Eat three bowls (with the bowl size a minimum of two cups) of a variety of vegetables with beans, plus three tablespoons of fermented foods a day.
6. Eat a cup of blueberries every day.

7. Pay attention to how you feel after each meal. How do you feel within the first two hours after you eat your food? Your body is the expert. Listen to it.
8. Make your dressings and sauces at home in batches, and store in the freezer if possible and desirable.
9. Read the ingredient labels of every single packaged product you use.
10. Prepare your food at 320 degrees Fahrenheit or lower. Steam, sauté, bake, and pressure cook with water and healthy fats.
11. Eat take-out or restaurant food no more than once a week.
12. Fast overnight for fourteen to sixteen hours regularly.

A Healthy Future Is Right in Front of You

To transform your health, you first need to develop the right habits. Every bite, every meal, is another step toward reaching the lifestyle you've dreamed about.

I know habits are hard to break. Trust me, I know it's not easy. I was raised with guilt if I didn't finish everything on my plate and wanted to throw food away. I was made to believe I had to eat often because my glucose was too low. But I discovered I was eating the wrong foods, and my glucose was spiking and dropping. I was metabolically inflexible, which got me stuck in a vicious cycle of constant eating because I had low energy and felt hungry every two hours.

Thankfully, I searched for answers until I discovered how to resolve the problem. But even though I've come a long way since my youth, I'm far from perfect. I still struggle with eating more than I need. Don't pressure yourself to be perfect; just take it one day at a time.

When trying to change your behavior, be sure to have a great strategy in place. I hope my ideas can inspire you to a life full of energy, joy, and vitality—because that's what you deserve.

If you eat real, whole foods, you won't crave junk food or feel like you're restricting yourself and sacrificing anything. You'll be able to enjoy a bite of dessert or a glass of wine on rare occasions and still feel great. You'll understand and feel the gains from eating real, whole foods and drinking clean water.

Helpful Glossary of Food Terms

Pasture-raised: An animal that's free to roam in a natural environment and eat grass, plants, bugs, and any other food their bodies are naturally adapted to digest.

Grass-fed: An animal that eats grass.

Grass-finished: An animal that is raised to maturity on only grass.

Pasteurization: The process of heating dairy to 160 degrees Fahrenheit for 15 seconds to eliminate microbes and other potentially harmful bacteria.

Raw/unpasteurized: Unheated other than the animal's natural body temperature, which is typically around 100 degrees Fahrenheit.

Free-range: A bird that's allowed to roam freely outdoors at least 51 percent of its life.

Cage-free: A bird that's not caged and thus free to roam.

Wild: Fish that are 100 percent wild.

Wild-caught: Fish that are caught in the wild and could have been spawned or lived part of their life on a fish farm.

Farmed: Fish that are kept in pens, tanks, or ponds.

Blue label: The most sustainable and environmentally friendly seafood.

CHAPTER THREE

TRANSFORMING YOUR ENERGY THROUGH SLEEP

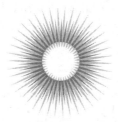

Most people are happy with a good family and a steady job. Indeed, those two elements provide a solid foundation for a happy life. But poor sleep can get in the way of enjoying that foundation to its fullest. That's what happens when you're tired all the time. This was the issue facing Kelly. She was tired every day, no matter what she did. Things got so bad, she started to have anxiety about not being able to sleep, which in turn made things even worse. When I evaluated Kelly, I discovered that she had an inconsistent sleep routine and eating schedule. She went to bed anywhere between 10:00 p.m. and midnight, and her sleep was interrupted all night. She would get up anywhere from 6:00 a.m. to 9:00 a.m. Kelly drank coffee in the late afternoon and snacked late at night—both a no-no if you want high-quality sleep and a healthy life.

Kelly's biggest challenges were that her habits were not aligned with her biology—the circadian rhythm we all need to understand and follow if we want to feel and function our best. Working together, I helped Kelly develop a consistent routine following the natural biological cycle. Within a few days, her habits changed, and she was able fall asleep easier and stay asleep throughout the night.

Now, Kelly wakes up feeling refreshed. She's committed to being in bed by 10:30 p.m., and she wakes up without an alarm clock at 6:30 a.m. And because of improved sleep, Kelly also eats better.

Every single client I work with has a dysregulated circadian rhythm—not by choice, but due to a lack of knowledge. We've touched on the fact that the circadian rhythm is your body's internal clock that operates on a roughly twenty-four-hour cycle. It regulates physiological processes, including sleep-wake cycles, hormone release, body temperature, and digestion. This internal clock is influenced by light and darkness, helping your body anticipate and adapt to changes in the environment.

A well-regulated circadian rhythm is crucial for overall health. Disruptions to your circadian rhythm can lead to sleep disorders, increased stress, metabolic issues, and a higher risk of chronic diseases.

As soon as my clients understand this system, it becomes easier for them to change their habits, and they quickly begin to feel better. That's because they understand *why* they need to change.

The Joy of Sleep

Better sleep equals a better mood, a better mood equals better health, and better health equals a better life. This all leads to greater joy.

Did you know that every ache, every extra pound of weight, and every disease can be connected to poor sleep issues? Your mood, focus, food cravings, metabolism, immune system, movement, relationships, and every single aspect of your life are all tied to the quality, quantity, and timing of your sleep.

The good news is that you can transform the way you think about sleep. That's essential, as sleep is one of life's most essential and rejuvenating activities. You may think you sleep just fine, but when your sleep improves, you'll recognize what you have been missing.

Get ready to embark on a journey that improves your overall health and wellness.

Activity: Self-Assessment of Your Day

1. During the day, do you find yourself struggling to keep your eyes open?
2. Are you unable to think clearly throughout the day?
3. Do you seek caffeine or medication just to make it through the day until bedtime?
4. Do you find yourself constantly irritable?
5. Are you unable to focus on even the simplest of tasks?
6. Are you often jumping from one thing to the next without accomplishing anything?
7. Are you too exhausted to exercise?
8. At the end of the day, do you find yourself resorting to alcohol or sleep medication to sedate you?

9. Do you spend sleepless nights worrying about what the future holds?
10. Do you need an alarm clock to wake you up most days of the week?

If you answered "yes" to any of the above questions, reflect on how often these situations occur: occasionally, frequently, nearly every day? Understanding your patterns can help identify the severity of your sleep dysregulation.

Sleep is not just about recharging your batteries. It is not just a passive state of rest. Sleep is an active process of repairing and rejuvenating our bodies. Every cell in the body, from our immune system to our gut to our brain, needs the healing power of sleep to work properly.

Sleep: A Nonnegotiable Necessity

Just like the sun goes down every day, we go to sleep every night. And we need that sleep so we can restore every part of our bodies, which allows us to perform fully again the next day.

What prevents us from getting the sleep we need? Sometimes we are like toddlers who want to continue playing with our favorite toy, be it scrolling on our phone or watching our favorite show.

Since we have the ability to delay sleep, we think we can do it again and again and again. But staying up late to watch TV, scroll endlessly through social media, or return work emails sacrifices our quality of sleep. More importantly, we damage our bodies at a cellular level.

We must understand that optimal sleep is necessary and natural; we're supposed to be fully rested. Developing correct sleep habits is as important as learning to eat the right whole foods and exercise regularly if we want to live well.

Fortunately, it's never too late to start learning. So, let's go!

The Domino Effect of Poor Sleep

We are complex beings. If you lack sleep, your food choices will be poor and your exercise will be compromised. In short, everything will be out of order and your health will suffer.

And yet, we all seem to pay the least attention to sleep's role in our vitality. We tend to focus on nutrition and exercise, but the reality is that lack of proper sleep is a serious problem affecting millions of people. According to research, about one in three adults does not get the recommended amount of uninterrupted sleep necessary to live well.[62]

Lack of sleep is a serious problem. It increases inflammation, which accelerates aging and leads to unwanted symptoms and diseases. Poor sleep damages every system from the immune system, to the cardiovascular system, to our brain's health system. When you're not fully rested, it's harder to learn and remember information, and more challenging to regulate blood sugar levels.

Studies show that if you only sleep for five hours for four nights in a row and measure your blood sugar, your test results will look the same as someone who has prediabetes.[63] This means your insulin hormone is dysregulated by poor sleep, and your response to carbohydrate-rich foods is the same as someone who has insulin resistance, prediabetes, or type 2 diabetes.

Four hours of sleep in one night lowers the activity of natural killer cells by about 70 percent.[64] These cells are a crucial part of our immune system, since they identify toxins and play a huge role in protecting against developing cancer.[65]

Research shows your cardiovascular system also suffers.[66] Losing one hour of sleep in the springtime leads to a 24 percent increase in heart attacks the next day. In the fall, when we gain one hour of sleep, people tend to have fewer heart attacks.[67]

You increase your risk for all causes of mortality by not prioritizing the quality, quantity, and timing of your sleep.

Not only the hormone insulin but all other hormones get out of whack with lack of proper sleep. The stress hormone cortisol tends to dip at night, but if you don't get enough rest, cortisol may remain elevated. When you sleep, your body also produces balanced amounts of ghrelin and leptin, two hormones that impact appetite and satiety.[68] If you don't get enough sleep (or your sleep is poor quality), you may produce too much ghrelin. That can indirectly lead to higher glucose levels by prompting you to overeat. Have you noticed that when you are sleep-deprived, you often crave more food, especially sweets and starches?

No pun intended, it's time for you to wake up. Sleep is the best free health investment you can make to live well.

Start by writing down your sleep routine so you can see exactly what it looks like and where you can improve for your health goals. Write down the answers to these questions:
- What is the first thing you do when you wake up?
- What do you do during that first awake hour of the morning?
- What time do you wake up in the morning?

- What time do you go to bed?
- What do you do in that final hour of the day to prepare for sleep?

The answers will tell you a lot about what you may need to change.

Come into My Bedroom

A few years ago, my husband started snoring and tossing and turning a lot more than before. The sounds and movements were waking me up and interrupting my sleep. Due to me being in perimenopause, with decreasing levels of progesterone, I was even more sensitive to noise, making it harder for me to fall back to sleep than before. Thirty to 40 percent of women between ages forty-five to fifty-five experience sleep disturbances during perimenopause. We become more sensitive to disturbances as our physiology changes. Without proper rest, I can't sustain my energy and focus throughout the day, I can't hit the gym as hard, and I'm not as patient. So I had to be honest about the changes we were both going through.

Since I like data, I measured my sleep with wearables. My Oura Ring and WHOOP heart rate monitor gave me a clear picture of how many times my sleep was disturbed and provided other valuable data like heart rate, temperature, and heart rate variability.

The solution was simple. We both understood the importance of a good night's sleep, so we decided to replace our king bed with two beds in the same room. I'm not disturbed by his movements anymore, and my husband now wears a nose strip and mouth tape to control the snoring. There was an immediate improvement in my sleep. *Bam!* That was easy!

What Happens During Sleep

Imagine your brain as a busy office that processes information all day. It is a space where important decisions are made, projects are assigned, and tasks are managed.

So what happens to this space at night? Let's explore the various stages of sleep in a simplified form to understand the benefits that take place within the brain.

Falling Asleep: From Awake to Light Sleep

Think of the initial stage of falling asleep as the first sweep of cleaning an office at the end of a workday. It's a brief transition period between wakefulness and deeper sleep, where the brain starts to wind down and relax.

As the office lights dim, the cleanup crew begins their work, picking up papers, straightening desks, and tidying common areas. They ensure everything is in order before moving on to the deeper, more thorough cleaning tasks. This is akin to the theta-wave stage of sleep, marking the onset of light sleep that begins each sleep cycle. Theta waves occur at a frequency of four to eight hertz. Theta waves are associated with deep relaxation and meditation, making them essential for mental rest and recovery.

Non-REM Deep Sleep: Slow-Wave Sleep

From light sleep, we transition into non-REM (non-rapid eye movement) deep sleep, also referred to as slow-wave deep sleep, because it is characterized by slow waves. This is the only time your brain can finally take a break and take care of itself without supervising you. This is the big cleanup. This phase accounts for about 20 percent of your sleep.[69]

The real heavy cleanup happens now. Much like a cleanup crew in an office who roll up their sleeves to sanitize surfaces, tackle big messes, and use heavy machinery for deep cleaning, this sleep stage is crucial for physical repair and a healthy, strong immune system.

During deep sleep, your heart rate, breathing, and body temperature all decrease. Cerebrospinal fluid literally flushes out toxins, waste, and all the plaque correlated with Alzheimer's and other neurodegenerative diseases. The pituitary gland releases growth hormone, which is vital for maintaining muscle and bone health and supporting a healthy metabolism. Blood flow to muscles increases, facilitating bodily repairs.

This critical phase of non-REM deep sleep typically occurs early in the night around the hours of 11:00 p.m. and 2:00 a.m. Staying up past 11:00 p.m. may mean missing out on this essential deep cleaning, increasing your hunger and tendency to crave unhealthy foods the next day. Over time, skipping this stage can lead to accumulated toxins in the brain, causing inflammation and increasing the risk of chronic diseases.[70]

Interestingly, non-REM sleep is also when most sleepwalking episodes occur.

REM Sleep

After deep sleep, we go through light sleep again and then transition into the REM (Rapid Eye Movement) phase, which makes up about 25 percent of our total sleep time.

Imagine a special office crew arriving to organize the day's documents into neat folders and files.

During REM sleep, your brain actively sorts through memories, processes emotions, and consolidates information from both positive experiences and traumas encountered throughout the day. This is also the stage when your most vivid dreams occur. Importantly, no adrenaline or serotonin is released during this phase, resulting in temporary paralysis—essentially, your body's way of making sure you don't physically act out your dreams.[71]

REM sleep is crucial for rejuvenating the mind. It supports memory retention, mood stability, and emotional health, and enhances problem-solving abilities. During this stage, both respiration and heart rate quicken. Missing out on REM sleep means missing a vital opportunity for emotional healing and cognitive maintenance.[72]

What Goes On in the Night

Each cycle of sleep includes light sleep, non-REM, and REM, and each lasts about ninety minutes. Throughout the night, you cycle through these stages four to five times. Think of it like a nighttime office cleanup crew that rotates through different cleaning phases, ensuring everything is deeply cleaned, organized, and spotless by morning. These repeated cycles provide significant restoration for both your body and mind.

By adhering to the fundamentals of biology, you wake up to a clean, fresh, and organized "office" each morning, ready to be joyful and productive without fatigue, aches, pains, or extra weight. But disrupting this complex system with poor daily habits leaves your office messy and disorganized, to the point where it may eventually become unmanageable.

Consider what you miss out on when you don't sleep well. Isn't it remarkable how the body knows exactly what to do, when to do it, and how to heal if we just provide what it needs?

All the stages—light sleep, deep sleep, and REM sleep—are essential. While you're busy during the day, your body works at night to rebuild itself, restoring your brain, rebuilding your immunity, cleaning out toxins, and repairing and recovering.

No sleep means no repair. No repair leads to cell as well as microbiome damage, and this can lead to diseases. It's as simple as that.

Introducing the Circadian Rhythm

What regulates our sleep and wake cycle? Light. Light then regulates the release of hormones that regulate our sleep. The hormones cortisol and adrenaline rise in the morning to wake us up. The hormone melatonin is released from the pineal gland in the evening to make sure we fall asleep. Melatonin continues to be released through the night to keep us asleep.

We've discussed how our bodies operate like clocks on twenty-four-hour cycles—our circadian rhythm. These clocks are internal. Every organ has a clock, and every cell has a clock. Our master clock, known as the suprachiasmatic nucleus, or SCN, is the brain-specific center that regulates all the clocks. When light hits the eye, information is sent to this brain-specific center.[73]

Based on the light, the brain interprets this information about what time of day it is. From there, information is sent to the rest of the body, guiding us on when to eat, digest, and sleep. This all happens at certain times based on what information has been shared from light.

In other words, blue light is the primary signal that sets the circadian rhythm in the master clock. This influences the function of just about every cell and organ within the body, from hormone production to gastric secretions to neurotransmitter levels to cellular repair and more.

We are now exposed to extremely high amounts of blue light. From electronic devices to LED and fluorescent bulbs to lit-up light switches, we now have blue light with us 24-7. This is incredibly confusing to our bodies. As a result, we experience poor sleep quality and duration, increased glucose levels, and excess stress from sympathetic nervous system activity.

We have a built-in system to rest and work. The more we appreciate it and create our daily habits based on this biological system, the better we live.

Think about what one hour of sleep does to you when the time changes twice a year. It's like jet lag; your body is confused, your hormones are dysregulated, and you feel low energy, depressed, and anxious. Now everything is confused; it's complete chaos. No structure, no predictability.

And just like babies need structure and predictability, we also need it as adults. Yes, we can get away with a lot more when we are teenagers and young adults, but as we age, hormone production changes, and we need to listen to our biology if we want to feel good and function to our full potential. Every time we go against biology, we lose.

Different Chronotypes

Chronotypes are similar to your body's personal clock setting that influences when you prefer to sleep or be awake and active. It's like having an internal schedule that guides you to your peak performance times.

There are four different chronotypes with fun names I did not create:

- **Lions** love the morning light and are most energetic in the first half of the day.
- **Bears** follow the sun's rhythm, feeling most productive in the daylight hours, and prefer a good night's sleep when it's dark.
- **Wolves** are the night owls, finding their stride when most people are winding down.
- **Dolphins** might toss and turn, finding it hard to dive deep into sleep or stick to a regular sleep-wake cycle.[74]

Understanding your chronotype can be a game changer. It can help you work with your body's natural rhythm rather than against it, making sleep—and life—a whole lot smoother.

I am definitely a Lion. I like to get up early, around 5:00 a.m., and be asleep by 9:00 p.m.

What are you?

Good Sleep Starts in the Morning: The Vital Morning Routine

When you first wake up, your brain is in the alpha state, which is associated with relaxation, meditation, and creativity. This calm state of mind is where clarity emerges, helping you to solve problems effectively.[75]

Think of your brain as a cold engine in the morning; it needs to warm up gently.

Give yourself a chance to wake up calmly and allow yourself to set positive intentions for the day. I like to keep my eyes closed after I wake up and try to recall my dreams and go through them; then I say thank-you for the new day and set my intentions. This practice helps me better handle the coming day and all the stressors that may come my way.

If you start your day rushed and stressed, on your phone, or reading the news, you miss the chance to warm up your brain. As such, you throw yourself into the day on high alert with an activated sympathetic nervous system, straining both your brain and body.

I suggest to my clients to start to practice waking up without an alarm clock. It's important to wake up naturally rather than using an alarm clock, as studies show that waking up in the middle of the REM cycle can leave you feeling tired.[76] If you must use an alarm clock, opt for a soft, calm alarm sound to ease the waking process.

The Problem with Caffeine

From the moment you wake up, a molecule called *adenosine* in the central brain starts accumulating, which is a naturally relaxing metabolite of ATP—adenosine triphosphate (the energy our mitochondria produces). This is getting you ready for sleep in the evening. It builds up as you are awake and gradually grows as you get into the evening. The more adenosine you have, the sleepier you feel. Once you fall asleep, your adenosine levels fall back down.

If you drink any type of caffeinated drink, whether it's coffee, green tea, or something else, it's important to understand the following biochemistry: Caffeine molecules latch on to the same receptor as adenosine. But they don't latch on to activate them to create sleepiness. Instead, caffeine blocks the receptor from adenosine's ability to attach, while adenosine continues to be created in the brain. Accordingly, caffeine is an adenosine receptor blocker, not necessarily a stimulant. Where does all the adenosine go? It stays in your bloodstream, waiting for the receptors to be free so it can latch on to them.

As caffeine is being metabolized by your liver, the receptors finally become available to all the adenosine to latch on to the receptor. Now, instead of the natural gradual adenosine latching on to the receptors, it's an avalanche of all the buildup of adenosine. That's why we may feel a "crash" a few hours after we had our morning coffee. How do most of us solve it? Repeating the cycle by reaching for more coffee.

Another fact to keep in mind is that caffeine has a half-life of about six to eight hours or more, depending on your enzymatic activity for breaking down and eliminating caffeine. That means that approximately 50 percent of caffeine is metabolized in six to eight hours.[77] If you have a cup of coffee at noon, you still have a quarter of that caffeine in your brain at midnight.

Even if you sleep through the night, caffeine hinders the quality of that sleep. And without the deep sleep needed to restore your physiology, brain, and muscular system, you speed up the aging process and damage your body.

A Caffeine Experiment

Sleeping dehydrates you, since you go without water for all those hours.

After you wake up, first drink two to three glasses of clean water, then go outside, set an intention for the day, or read your vision for the day (more on this in the inner environment chapter).

Your body's cortisol levels naturally peak within the first hour after waking helping you feel alert and ready for the day. Consuming any caffeine during this peak cortisol period can reduce the effectiveness of caffeine because your body is already at its natural alertness peak. It makes no sense to add to it.

Enjoy your coffee an hour later. You may not even want it anymore.

This timing can help prevent the development of tolerance, which can actually make your morning cup more effective over time. Stop caffeine intake no later than noon so the body has time to metabolize it and remove it from your system.

Following these two simple caffeine steps will result in increased focus and energy.

Changing the caffeine habit may not be easy, I know. I used to have green tea in the morning and coffee around noon. I switched my coffee to matcha tea for more health benefits, but a few years into perimenopause, I wasn't feeling great. I then learned that caffeine could influence lowering one of the main thyroid hormones, T3, which my labs showed was decreasing. Low T3 can lead to hypothyroidism, which can lead to fatigue, weight gain, and other health challenges.[78] I have been feeling so much better after eliminating caffeine, and my T3 levels went back up within a short time. The only caffeine I get now is from cocoa powder or chocolate.

I replaced matcha tea with herbal teas or dandelion and chicory root powder. The dandelion and chicory drink smells like coffee. Try it. It's delicious. I quickly forgot about coffee. I feel much better without any caffeine.

Daytime: How About Napping?

Some people thrive on naps in the afternoon, and some people don't. I never napped until I reached perimenopause. Similarly, many of my clients have found that napping helps them. However, as we progress in our work together, and they adjust their daily habits and sleep better, the need for naps dissipates.

Naps can be great if your night sleep remains optimal. Studies show a 20 percent improvement in memory and learning just by napping.[79] Your emotional health improves as well. The problem with naps, however, is that they may decrease your quality of sleep at night. Pay attention to your night's sleep, and fix that before you start fixing it with naps.

I suggest listening to your body and wearing a tracker like a WHOOP or an Oura Ring. There may be times when you need a twenty- to thirty-minute nap. Sometimes I need twenty minutes of rest, and sometimes I just need to close my eyes for ten minutes while listening to calming sounds, and theta waves, or doing body scan exercises like yoga nidra. Especially during times when I spend hours studying and writing, my brain needs a little reboot.

When you feel your energy dip in the early afternoon, it is a completely normal biological process. I usually feel a dip in energy around 2:00 p.m. This dip, called *postprandial dip*, happens naturally anytime between 1:00 and 4:00 p.m. when your body temperature and blood glucose level drop and you feel more tired.[80]

When this happens, give your body a moment of rest. Find a quiet place or put headphones on and play recordings of theta-wave meditation music and close your eyes instead of reaching for stimulants or coffee. Shifting your mindset around this will create a stronger, lasting health.

TIP

1. A great time for a short nap is right after you learn something new, like reading a science study or learning a new song on a piano. Your brain will consolidate the new learning and you'll be able to understand and remember it better.
2. Another great time for a nap is when your body's temperature drops in the hours from 1–4 p.m..
3. After a nap, if you feel a little groggy, put your hands and face in ice-cold water and then go outside. You will feel refreshed and energized.

Dinnertime: How The Right Foods Can Improve Your Sleep

What you eat during the day can help you at night. Foods rich in potassium, prebiotics, tryptophan, and magnesium are easy to digest, making them perfect for promoting sleep. Taking it easy on heavy, fatty meals and avoiding too much protein (which supports the dopamine release we want during the day) may give you better sleep.

Low-carb foods (up to one hundred grams of carbs) seem to increase deep slow-wave sleep, while high-carbs foods tend to increase REM.[81] So, for example, if you measure your sleep and tend to have more deep sleep and less REM, you may experiment with adding some sweet potatoes or quinoa to your dinner plate and see how your sleep shifts.

Here are some foods I like to eat for dinner:

- Avocado
- Pumpkin seeds
- Almonds
- Leafy greens
- Yogurt
- Eggs
- Salmon
- Honey
- Kiwi
- Banana
- Root vegetables like carrots and celery root
- Collagen powder (high in glycine and great for detox-ification, which is what takes place in your body at night)

The Problem with Alcohol

It may feel like an alcoholic drink in the evening helps you get sleepy. But if you have alcohol in your system when going to sleep, you wake up through the night more than you may realize. These interruptions of your sleep suppress REM sleep. Alcohol also increases your heart rate, decreases the variability between heartbeats, and increases restlessness.

As mentioned earlier, sleep is dehydrating, and alcohol dehydrates as well. That's what causes the hangover.

But if you want to enjoy an occasional drink, experiment with these tips:

- Drink one glass of water with each glass of alcohol to hydrate.
- Drink early in the afternoon and no later than three hours before bed, just like with eating food, so your liver has some time to metabolize and eliminate the alcohol.
- Take complex minerals like magnesium, glycine, and alpha-lipoic acid to help your body detoxify after drinking. Glycine is an incredibly important, powerful amino acid with many different roles, mainly detoxification.

Remove Obstacles for Good Sleep

- Identify a snoring or tossing partner and make accommodations for separate beds.
- Remove disruptive sounds, which increase hormones like adrenaline and cortisol.
- Remove digital clocks and night lights.
- Eliminate alcohol and cigarette use.
- Avoid consuming caffeine after noon.
- Avoid intense exercise in the late afternoon.
- Avoid news, work, and difficult conversations that will stimulate stress one to two hours before bedtime

Winding Down: Falling Asleep Takes Preparation and Time

You don't get up in the morning and immediately do a 200-pound bench press, right? You must warm up before lifting heavy weights at the gym. We talked about warming up our brains in the morning, but the same concept applies to sleep. You need to fall into sleep gradually.

Could you just fall asleep anywhere, anytime in your teens? Probably. But that doesn't happen as we get older. We have to adjust our sleep routine based on many factors.

How to Get Naturally Great Sleep

Review this checklist for ideas on how you can plan ahead to improve your sleep.

Your Bedroom Environment

- **Add plants to your bedroom.** Plants add oxygen and offer a calming effect. Consider easy-to-care-for plants such as snake plants.
- **Check the humidity in your bedroom.** If the air is too dry, it is much harder to sleep.
- **Check your home's air filter.** Make sure you have clean air in your bedroom. Make sure your room is not filled with toxic air and mold.
- **Dust and vacuum regularly.** Implement a weekly routine of dusting and vacuuming your bedroom to help keep the air clean and free of toxins.
- **Set the right room temperature.** While you sleep, your body temperature will drop one degree. To support the body's natural process, your bedroom thermostat should not be set higher than 67 degrees Fahrenheit. I keep mine at 65 degrees.
- **Remove all electronics from your bedroom.** TVs, computers, and phones all have that tiny blue light that will disrupt your sleep and emit EMFs (electromagnetic fields). There is no space for these

electronics in the bedroom. Remember, the bedroom
is for sleep.

- **Get the necessary sleeping tools.** Consider having
mouth tape, nose snoring strips, and an eye mask on
your bedside table. Each of these can improve the
quality of your sleep.
- **Create a pitch-dark environment.** Use blackout
curtains that you can pull shut, or use tape or film
covers to make your windows black. Put electrical
tape over any/all indicator lights on electronics or
light switches.
- **Use red light bulbs.** Use these for all the lamps in
your house and turn those on in the evening, while
turning off all the overhead lights. Red light does not
affect your circadian rhythm, therefore it is the best
light to use at night
- **Evaluate what sounds you hear.** Is there excessive noise, such as street sounds, coming into your
bedroom? Other sounds? The volume of these sounds
can affect your sleep. Consider using earplugs.

Your Bed

- **Evaluate your mattress and pillow.** Do you wake
up with pain? Do you snore? Breathe heavy? It may
be due to your mattress or pillow. How old is your
mattress? What is your mattress made of? Ensure
your mattress is made of natural materials like cotton,
natural latex, or wool, with no synthetic materials or
fire retardants. A supportive, toxin-free mattress is
crucial for your health and sleep quality. Generally,
mattresses should be replaced every seven to ten

years, depending on the material and usage. How is your body alignment and posture? How is your pillow? Is your neck hurting when you get up? It may take a while, but keep hunting until you find the right pillow—it's worth the search. Also, consider if it is time to invest in an organic and more comfortable mattress. My favorite is the Naturepedic brand.

- **Evaluate your sheets.** Are your sheets clean, comfortable, and made of natural fabrics like bamboo, silk, cotton, or hemp? Do you wash them every week? As for your comforter, toss the down variety; it may be causing allergies. My preference is wool, organic cotton, or organic foam.

- **Evaluate your bed buddy.** Do you deal with a snoring person or a dog? How do you sleep when you sleep alone or in a different room in your house? Is it time for a separate bed or bedroom?

- **Consider mental associations.** Do you associate your bed with sleep? Do you sleep better in other rooms of the house or when you travel? If so, this may be because you have spent time on your phone when in bed or have not been able to sleep there for a while, and your brain now associates this place with anything other than sleep. To break this cycle, start by removing all electronic devices, including the TV, phones, and computers, from your bedroom. The bedroom should be for sleep, period. Additionally, try sleeping in another room for a few nights to reset your brain's associations. Once you've reestablished the connection between your bed and restful sleep, go back to your bedroom and start to associate it with sleep only. Your brain will get the message, and you will sleep deeply and peacefully again.

- **Sleep inclined.** About six inches of upper body elevation improves sleep. The elevation of the entire body leads to a natural remedy for snoring, lowering blood pressure, and increasing circulation.[82]

Your Daily Schedule

- **Keep a consistent schedule, including weekends.** The data is clear: You will be healthier if you pick one wake-up time and stick to it.[83] Go to bed and get up at the same time every day.
- **Exercise at the right time of day.** Exercise improves sleep quality. But be sure to engage in strenuous workouts in the morning or early afternoon. This helps to keep your body's core temperature lower when it's time to go to sleep.
- **Be in bed by 10:30 p.m.** To get enough deep sleep, you need to observe and respect your body's biological clock and circadian rhythm by going to bed on the early side.

The Problem with Sleep Medication

Many people use antihistamines like Benadryl (with the active ingredient diphenhydramine) as a sleep aid, but this can be a dangerous habit. A 2016 study published in *JAMA Neurology* found that long-term use of anticholinergic drugs, such as diphenhydramine, is linked to an increased risk of dementia, including Alzheimer's disease.[84]

To be sure, Benadryl and similar medications are not meant to improve your sleep. Rather, they make you unconscious—that's a big difference. So they are not solving the cause of *why* you are not sleeping well. They are only creating bigger problems and possible dependency.

Using sleep aids once in a while for travel or during higher amounts of stress may be necessary. However, before you turn to medication, talk to your functional medicine practitioner to help you identify the reasons and find other options.

Screen for Sleep Disorders

Do you have sleep apnea? This is a serious issue that must be addressed. You can test for this with an app at home, but it's best to talk to a trusted functional medicine doctor.

Going Deeper for a Good Night's Sleep

We've talked about how enjoying a good night's sleep begins from the moment you wake up until you return to your bed at night. This section takes a deeper look at how you can prepare to get the most out of your dedicated sleep time.

Going through your regular daily schedule in your mind, and as a review, look at each of these sections and consider which steps you could take to implement better habits and routines into your daily life. Your will feel better, function better, and create great health.

Morning Routine

When you wake up, stay in bed for a few minutes while your eyes are closed. Spend time processing your dreams and setting yourself up for a great day with good thoughts.

Think good thoughts. These are just some suggestions; you can make up your own consistent habits that work for you:

- Thank you for this day.
- Today is a good day.
- Every day, in every way, my life is better and better.
- I am grateful for ...

Start Your Day with the WISE Routine

- **W is for Water.** Begin your morning by drinking two to three glasses of purified water. Throughout the night, your body works to remove waste from your organs, and hydrating first thing in the morning helps flush these toxins out. *Tip*: Keep a thirty-two-ounce water bottle on your nightstand so it's ready for you when you wake up.
- **I is for Intention.** Set a positive intention for your day. As you sip your water, take a moment to reflect on how you want to feel and what you'd like to accomplish. This can help ground you and align your focus.
- **S is for Sunlight.** Get ten to twenty minutes of sunlight before 9:00 a.m. to set your circadian rhythm. Step outside or, if it's too cold, stand by a window and let natural light into your eyes. Even on a cloudy day, outdoor light is powerful. If it's still dark when you wake up, turn on an overhead light, and head outside as soon as the sun rises.
- **E is for Exercise.** Move your body with gentle stretching, a ten-minute yoga session, or a walk. This helps stimulate your lymphatic system, improves circulation, and loosens your joints for the day ahead.

By following the WISE routine daily—Water, Intention, Sunlight, Exercise—you'll set yourself up for a day of energy, focus, and well-being.

Three Essential Habits Before Bed for Restful Nights

1. **Stop eating food.** You'll recall from our chapter on food that production of digestive enzymes, as well as insulin, decreases as the sun goes down. Your dinner at 6:00 p.m. is being digested until about 11:00 p.m. If you eat close to bedtime, your body is forced to digest the food, which interrupts the process of sleep. As such, you have two tasks competing to get completed at once, so nothing gets done 100 percent. Eat as early as possible.

2. **Regulate your body's temperature.** A hot shower, bath, or sauna can temporarily raise your body's surface temperature. The heat helps you vasodilate on the surface of the skin, or helps your blood vessels widen, and all the heat forces the body to cool you down. This heat exposure is followed by a decrease in your body's core temperature, which can help facilitate sleep. We fall asleep more easily when our core temperature drops slightly.

3. **Block blue light.** We need a faucet full of melatonin. Blue light makes the faucet turn off or drip slowly, which is not good. The blue light from your phone, TV, and lights in the house suppresses melatonin production. In fact, a study shows that kids who are exposed to bright light an hour before bed have melatonin levels suppressed by 88 percent (it's 50 percent for

adults).[85] This suppression creates fragmented sleep, which impacts your ability to fall asleep and go into deep sleep.

If you must look at screens at night, wear high-quality blue-light blockers that block all blue light—these should have a dark orange lens. I recommend you find a reputable company like TrueDark, Ra Optics, or Swanwick Sleep.

Habits for One Hour Before Going to Bed

When preparing for sleep, the overall goal is to get the parasympathetic nervous system in a calm mode. And it's important to be consistent with your routine, because our brains like routines.

1. **Turn off all overhead lights.** Shut off your TV, computer, and phone. Turn on lamps with installed red or yellow light bulbs. Red light has a longer wavelength and lower energy compared to blue light, making it less likely to interfere with sleep-inducing melatonin production.
2. **Play music.** Just like when we were kids and were lucky enough to have our caregivers sing us lullabies, music calms the nervous system. Music gives the brain something else to focus on instead of ruminating thoughts.
3. **Lower stress.** Eliminate negativity, be it from the news, difficult conversations with your partner, and other stress-inducing sources.
4. **Focus on gratitude.** Write down three "wins" you had during the day. These can be any positive achievement. I do this with my family every night—we share

our wins with one another. This practice makes you focus on the positives before sleep. Life can be challenging, so focus on at least one thing to feel good about before sleep.

5. **Body scan.** Practice progressive muscle relaxation where you tense and release your muscles progressively from the tips of your toes to the top of your head. Listening to a guided yoga nidra body scan is also a great way to calm the mind.

6. **Create a scent.** Use a few drops of lavender and/or ylang-ylang essential oil on your pillow. The scent relaxes the muscles in the body. I put a few drops on my pillow every night.

7. **Unwind with joy.** Enjoy a relaxing time reading a good book, taking a gentle stroll, or spending quiet time with your pet. Let go of the day.

Do You Have Physical Pain?

If you are dealing with pain that's preventing you from having a good night's sleep, talk to a trusted functional medicine practitioner, osteopath, or physical therapist. Try acupuncture, massage, or other release techniques from qualified professionals.

Consider Supplements for Better Sleep

While supplements can be helpful, they do not fix problems entirely; they are only one aspect of a healthy sleep routine. I've found these supplements to be beneficial:

- *Magnesium Malate and Glycinate.* Magnesium is one of the most important minerals, yet many have a deficiency in it. Magnesium promotes relaxation and sleep.
- *PS 100 (phosphatidylserine)* lowers nighttime cortisol.
- *Ashwagandha* clears out cortisol from the receptors, so I take it before bed and cycle it, which means taking it for two weeks and then taking a week off.
- *Glycine* calms the nervous system, supports the liver's detoxification process, and induces vasodilation throughout the body to promote lowering of core body temperature.
- *Collagen powder* mixed with water is high in glycine. It's another option to supplement with glycine and get the benefits of improved skin, joint, and tissue health.
- *Raw honey* raises liver glycogen to stabilize your glucose at night if you are waking up because of big dips in glucose. Try taking a teaspoon full before bed.
- *Valerian, hops, passionflower, and chamomile* tinctures may be helpful.

For any other suggestions on supplements, please consult your functional medicine practitioner.

Seven to nine quality hours of consistent sleep is the foundation of good health, influencing everything from our hormonal health to our heart health to our mental health. Prioritizing a consistent sleep routine and creating an environment that supports deep, restorative sleep is one of the most powerful steps you can take for your overall well-being. Remember, quality sleep isn't a luxury—it's a necessity for living well and thriving every day. Come back to this chapter as often as you need to, using the tips and insights to help you build lasting habits that will transform your sleep and health.

CHAPTER FOUR

BUILDING STRONG HEALTH THROUGH MOVEMENT

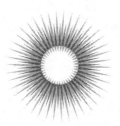

Dan poured his heart and soul into his work. Nights, weekends, holidays—every moment was devoted to growing his business. As a single man, he had the flexibility to prioritize his career above all else, and by society's standards he was thriving.

But behind the facade of success, Dan's relentless work ethic came at a significant cost. By his forties, he found himself overweight, constantly fatigued, and reliant on sugary snacks and drinks to get through the day. His weekend mornings were spent in bed as long as possible, and his evenings were lost in a haze of TV shows. When prescribed statins, the side effects proved unbearable, pushing him to think more seriously about his lifestyle.

Dan knew a change was necessary, but the thought of taking the first step felt so overwhelming. He had no idea where to even begin, so it was easier to just not change anything at all. Exercise had been absent from his life since high school, and the idea of moving again felt daunting.

Then, everything shifted. When we began working together, I helped Dan understand his body better and feel more empowered to embrace a healthier lifestyle. We started with simple changes: better eating habits, improved sleep routines, and gentle, consistent exercise. Initially, Dan took short walks around his neighborhood, slowly increasing his daily activity. He hired a trainer who guided him through safe, basic exercises at the gym.

Within a year, Dan's transformation was nothing short of remarkable. He shed the excess fat, built muscle, and regained his stamina. Hiking trails became his new passion, and he no longer needed medication. His commitment to daily movement revitalized not just his body, but also his mind and spirit.

Now, at fifty-five, Dan feels phenomenal. He lifts weights, jumps rope, and pedals away on the assault bike two days a week. While TV still has its place, Dan now values movement and health above all—an achievement that surpasses any business success.

In this chapter, I emphasize that daily movement is nonnegotiable. Just like our food choices, variety and balance in exercise are essential. We can't confine ourselves to one type of exercise for an hour a day and remain idle for the rest. Movement must be a constant in our lives, a vital part of our journey to health and happiness.

When We Stop Moving, We Stop Living

No matter how tired I feel in the morning, working out always lifts my spirits and boosts my energy. It might seem counterintuitive that exercise can energize you when you're tired, but it all comes down to our body's amazing messengers—hormones.

When we exercise, our bodies releases hormones like cortisol, adrenaline, noradrenaline, and endorphins. These powerful molecules give you messages of alertness, energy, and better mood, transforming fatigue into vitality and joy.

We are supposed to move, so it makes sense that we feel so much better when we do any form of movement. Whatever your "why" is, as long as it pulls you to move, just do it. Only thirty minutes of higher intensity exercise—a brisk walk, a bike ride, weight lifting—will elevate your mood and boost your energy for the rest of the day.

Exercise is also important because we need to build and maintain muscle mass. If you don't use it, you lose it. If you don't use your muscles, you lose the muscles. Ongoing physical inactivity has serious consequences. Can you get up from the ground without using your hands? Take your overhead luggage and place it in the overhead airplane storage? Can you open a jar? Pick up and carry bags of groceries? Push the vacuum cleaner?

All these daily tasks require muscles, flexibility, and balance. If we stop using our muscles as we age, we are lowering our quality of life and length of life—by choice.

Being strong allows you to support your body in various situations and positions. We have to work on building and maintaining muscle strength throughout our lifetime. Be honest with yourself and assess how much, and how well, you move daily.

The Hard Facts About Muscle Loss

Adults lose between 3 to 8 percent of muscle mass per decade after the age of thirty. This rate of muscle loss accelerates significantly after the age of sixty.[86] This muscle degradation, called *sarcopenia*, significantly impacts strength, mobility, and overall health. Do not take this lightly.

Sarcopenia significantly impacts quality of life and health outcomes in older adults. Regular strength training and proper nutrition are essential for maintaining muscle mass, and function as we age.[87]

Movement Is as Essential as Sleep

Movement is one of the most important activities you do daily. Just like consistent sleep, consistent movement is crucial for health and longevity. You wouldn't stop sleeping simply because you didn't feel like it. The same applies to consistent movement or exercise.

But movement isn't just about avoiding sedentariness; it's about enhancing every facet of bodily function, from the lymphatic system's role in immunity to regulating metabolic processes, to brain and heart function.

Think of your body like a car. If a car is left sitting in a garage, not driven for months or years, the battery will die, the tires will deflate, and the engine oil will degrade. When you finally need to use the car, it won't even start.

Similarly, when we lead a sedentary lifestyle, our bodies are like unused cars. Muscles atrophy and lose strength due to lack of use. Joint lubrication diminishes, you become stiff, and every movement hurts. Your physical functions decline or, even worse, fall apart.

Engaging in physical activities daily, such as lifting weights, walking, and stretching, helps maintain muscle mass, joint health, and overall body function. Starting these habits as early as possible is like opening your savings account at a young age and making regular deposits: The savings build up with time. Doing one deposit a year is not going to provide much return on investment.

Even if you've been sedentary for years, beginning to move and challenge your body can revive it quickly. Start small, be consistent, and gradually increase the intensity of your activities to challenge and grow your body.

Many people stop engaging in exercise as they start getting older. When we stop using type II muscle fibers (responsible for short bursts of power and speed in movements like jumping), which are crucial for performing many daily tasks efficiently, we increase the probability of falls and injuries. As we age, maintaining balance and quick reflexive muscle responses is vital for preventing falls.

Here are some helpful examples of exercises to maintain the health of these muscles:

- Sprints that last from ten to thirty seconds
- Box jumps
- Plyometric exercises like push-ups
- Medicine ball slams (lifting a heavy medicine ball above your head and then forcefully slamming it down engages multiple muscle groups in fast-twitch fiber activation—the muscle that contracts fast under force, like sprinting or jumping)
- Jump rope
- Battle ropes (making waves with heavy ropes in a rapid, explosive manner for short durations is great for upper-body, fast-twitch muscle engagement)
- Tennis, pickleball, dance, and ping-pong

Use that incredible body you have, and use it safely and regularly throughout the day.

The Dangers of a Sedentary Lifestyle

A sedentary lifestyle is now recognized as being as dangerous as smoking and excessive alcohol consumption. Think about it: When you sit, you use minimal muscle to hold yourself up. It takes long, consistent work to grow and maintain strength. This can't be done quickly over a short period; it takes daily, lifelong dedication.

Research indicates that prolonged sitting can increase the risk of heart disease, diabetes, and even cancer. For instance, people who sit for long periods have a 147 percent higher risk of suffering a heart attack or stroke and a 112 percent higher risk of developing diabetes.[88]

Even if you exercise every day for one hour, long periods of inactivity for the rest of the day can negate many of the benefits of exercise.[89] Obviously, that one hour is absolutely better than no exercise at all, though understand that you still will be at higher risk of developing diseases than someone who moves regularly throughout the day. The human body is designed to move, and when we remain sedentary, our metabolism slows down and we burn fewer calories, leading to weight gain and increased fat accumulation around vital organs, called *visceral fat*. This is the fat we can't see, but we can measure with tools like the DEXA scan, which I've mentioned in previous chapters. Visceral fat can exacerbate insulin resistance and other metabolic disorders.

Simple changes like standing up every thirty to forty-five minutes, taking walking breaks, or doing jumping jacks, push-ups, or squats can make a significant difference in your heart health and overall well-being.

The Connection Between Movement and Lymphatic Fluid

Moving is important for removing toxins. The lymphatic system helps get rid of toxins. Blood is pumped through the body by the heart, but the lymphatic system does not have a pump; it doesn't move unless we move, and it doesn't remove waste unless we move. It relies on the movement of our muscles to circulate the toxins out.

Exercise is crucial for managing your blood sugar and glucose levels. When you're active, your muscles act like engines that need fuel, using glucose from your bloodstream as a quick source of energy. Normally, your body stores glucose in the liver and muscles (called glycogen), which can be quickly converted back to glucose when needed, like during exercise or a stressful activity, or even an argument.

During movement, muscles first use the glucose from the blood. But they also use other energy sources, including stored glycogen and fatty acids. The relative contribution of blood glucose depends on factors like exercise intensity and duration.

Insulin helps by acting like a key, opening your cells so glucose can enter them more easily. Low-intensity exercising, especially after meals, helps prevent spikes in blood sugar because muscles use glucose more efficiently, thanks to an increase in glucose transporters type 4 (GLUT4) on their surfaces. This means less insulin is needed.

GLUT4 is a protein made from a specific sequence of amino acids that fold into a unique structure, giving it the ability to respond to insulin signaling.[90] GLUT4 acts as a special door inside your muscle cells and fat cells. When the

GLUT4 door is closed, glucose can't easily enter the muscle and stays in the bloodstream, which can cause problems.

So, what opens the door? Glad you asked!

When insulin, a signaling hormone, reaches the muscle cell, it binds to receptors on the cell surface. This triggers a series of signals inside the cell that move the stored GLUT4 doors to the cell walls, allowing glucose to enter the muscle cell. This is exactly what we want—glucose in the muscle, not the bloodstream where it could be stored as fat.

And guess what else opens the door? Exercise!

When you exercise, these GLUT4 doors move to the cell surface, helping your muscles grab glucose to use as energy. This process lowers blood sugar levels by pulling sugar out of the blood and into the muscles where it's needed.

What increases the number of GLUT4 doors? Regular exercise! The more you exercise, the more GLUT4 doors you have, making your body better at controlling blood sugar over time. The more muscle you have, the more GLUT4 doors you have, leading to less glucose in the bloodstream—reducing inflammation and the risk of disease. Pretty amazing, right?

So, to sum it up: The more you lift weights and build muscle, the more GLUT4 doors you have in your muscle cells to use glucose from your food, lowering your chances of developing type 2 diabetes or other metabolic diseases caused by overconsumption of sugar and simple carbs.

Training for Young Mitochondria

Mitochondria become less efficient as we age. There are two important exercise types to incorporate into your weekly routine to increase mitochondrial volume and produce more healthy, young mitochondria. (Refer back to the mitochondria section in the introduction as a refresher.)

Zone 2 Training

Exercise scientists classify movement into the five zones of exercise. Zone 1 is the lowest intensity, like doing chores around your house, and zone 5 is the highest intensity, at your maximum heart rate.[91] Zone 2 exercises are great because they're fairly easy to do and increase your heart health and fat oxidation. Zone 2 training includes activities like a fast, steady walk, bike ride, or rowing movement where you do not create much lactate; you are in the fat-burning zone (fat oxidation).

Lactate is a byproduct of anaerobic metabolism, and it is made during high-intensity exercise when the oxygen demand exceeds the supply and the body breaks down glucose into lactate for rapid bursts of energy. Simply put, when your lactate levels go up, you are in a glucose-burning state and are not burning fat.

Zone 2 exercise is aerobic training: You're working at 60 to 70 percent of your maximum heart rate. The recommendation is 150 minutes of moderate-intensity exercise per week, which is supported by numerous health organizations, including the American Heart Association and the World Health Organization.[92] Studies show that this amount of exercise significantly reduces the risk of chronic diseases such as heart disease, stroke, diabetes, and some cancers.[93]

Regular zone 2 training increases the efficiency of the heart and lungs, improving blood flow and oxygen supply to the tissues. This intensity level optimizes the body's ability to use fat as a fuel source. Zone 2 training stimulates the production of mitochondria in muscle cells, enhancing endurance and overall energy levels.

Because zone 2 training is not overly strenuous, it helps reduce cortisol levels and does not overly tax the body, making it sustainable and beneficial for long-term health.

I walk on the treadmill three to four times a week for sixty minutes on a level-five incline and speed of three to three and a half miles per hour, while spending the time reading or listening to audiobooks or a podcast. Remember, proper exercise is about consistency and doing this for the rest of your life, so I hope you fall in love with this routine.

High-Intensity Interval Training (HIIT)

HIIT is vigorous training that creates a high demand for rapid energy. Opposite to zone 2 training, during intense exercises, the body uses glucose to then produce lactate as an immediate fuel source. Unlike glucose, lactate can be utilized more efficiently during high-demand situations because it bypasses the complex energy production processes in the mitochondria that glucose goes through to create energy. This means you get instant energy from lactate; it's fast when you need it.

Lactate is incredibly important for energy; it is also a signaling molecule. That means lactate signals, or sends messages to, other cells, affecting the glucose transporter protein mentioned above. Every time you do HIIT, lactate levels increase, and the lactate triggers GLUT4 to enhance the transport of glucose from the bloodstream into the muscle cells. Pretty amazing, right?[94]

Lactate also signals your body to produce more PGC-1alpha (peroxisome proliferator-activated receptor gamma coactivator 1-alpha). This substance plays a crucial role in how our cells manage energy. It helps increase the number of mitochondria (mitochondrial biogenesis) and function of mitochondria in the muscle and brain. This is important because a high amount of healthy mitochondria means unstoppable daily energy. The rise in lactate also boosts the production of BDNF (brain-derived neurotrophic factor), which supports brain health, cognitive function, and even memory.[95]

PGC-1alpha also helps our bodies generate heat in brown adipose tissue (a process called thermogenesis) in response to cold and manage its internal temperature. Brown adipose tissue (BAT), or brown fat, contains more mitochondria than white fat. BAT generates heat to maintain body temperature, especially in cold environments. It burns energy through a process called non-shivering thermogenesis. PGC-1alpha activates proteins in brown fat to convert calories into heat, unlike white fat, which stores energy. PGC-1alpha supports our cells in dealing with oxidative stress by boosting antioxidant levels, protecting our cells from damage. PGC-1alpha regulates gluconeogenesis in the liver and glucose uptake in muscle.

And let's not forget about the microbiome, because exercise plays a significant role in shaping the gut microbiome, the diverse community of microorganisms living in our intestines. Regular physical activity has been shown to enhance the diversity and abundance of beneficial bacteria.[96] This increase in microbial diversity helps improve digestion, enhance immune function, and reduce inflammation.

Recent studies show that exercise leads to an increase in beneficial butyrate-producing bacteria.[97] Butyrate is fatty acid produced by gut bacteria. Butyrate has anti-inflammatory properties, may prevent cancer, speeds up metabolism, and reduces inflammation.[98] Due to the gut-brain connection, exercise promotes better mental health by reducing stress and anxiety, which in turn positively affects gut health.

The Norwegian Exercise

There are many types of HIIT exercises, though one of my favorites is the Norwegian exercise, because its benefits are supported by strong research conducted by Norwegian scientists at the Norwegian University of Science and Technology (NTNU) in Trondheim, Norway.[99] Thus, the name!

The Norwegian exercise, also known as the Norwegian 4x4, is simple and effective, yet challenging. It's designed to improve cardiovascular health, increase aerobic capacity, and enhance overall fitness.

Here's how the Norwegian 4x4 exercise works:

- **High intensity:** Perform four minutes of high-intensity exercise, such as running, rowing, or cycling, at 85 to 95 percent of your maximum heart rate. This intensity should feel challenging.
- **Recovery phase:** Follow each high-intensity phase with three to four minutes of active, low-intensity recovery. This allows your heart rate to decrease and prepares your body for the next high-intensity interval.
- **Repeat:** Complete four cycles of the high-intensity and recovery phases.

Cool down and enjoy the benefits of every single organ in your body getting healthier.

Regularly performing 4x4 intervals can increase your VO2 max, which is the maximum amount of oxygen your body can use during exercise, a key indicator of cardiovascular fitness.

I have this exercise on my calendar once a week. Grab your calendar and schedule it for this week.

Muscles Are a Necessity for a Healthy Life

Muscle mass keeps you from tripping, falling, and breaking bones. Frailty and dementia go up, and quality of life goes down tremendously, as muscle mass goes down.

Muscle mass is directly correlated with health and longevity. Strong muscles support strong bones and joints, helping to prevent injuries and degenerative bone conditions like osteoporosis. As we age, healing from falls and fractures becomes more challenging, making it essential to maintain healthy bones and muscles through resistance training.

Muscle is metabolically active tissue; it demands energy for every cellular function, even when you are resting and sitting. Think of your muscles as little engines in your body that are always running, even when you're just sitting or resting. These engines need fuel to keep going, which means they burn calories even when you're not moving.

As we age or lead a sedentary lifestyle, we tend to lose muscle, which is like turning off some of those engines. When this happens, your body needs less fuel, and your basal metabolic rate (BMR)—the number of calories your body needs to keep basic functions like breathing and circulation going—starts to drop. The less muscle you have, the fewer calories you burn at rest.

So keeping your muscles strong is like keeping your body's engine running efficiently, helping you maintain a higher metabolism even when you're not actively exercising.

Imagine this: Each pound of muscle you have burns about six calories daily at rest. As such, if you lose five pounds of muscle because you are not lifting weights, you will burn approximately thirty fewer calories daily when resting; some studies suggest even fifty fewer calories.[100]

It may not seem like much, but over time, this gradually adds up to lower daily energy needs, making it easier to gain fat and harder to lose it with less muscle. This is just one example of why muscle is so important for metabolism.

Higher muscle mass is associated with a lower risk of developing all diseases! Muscle acts as a glucose sink; it helps remove glucose from the blood and stores it for later use. The great news is that your body can tolerate more carbohydrates with more skeletal muscle!

How to Build Muscle

Weight-bearing exercises alone won't build muscle unless supported by eating real, whole, protein-rich foods. Similarly, food alone can't build muscle unless you also engage in resistance training. When you combine the right type, frequency, and intensity of exercise with healthy, protein-rich foods, you can build and maintain muscle mass throughout your life.

During exercise, muscles experience microtears that need to be repaired with amino acids, the building blocks of proteins. This process allows muscles to rebuild and grow during recovery.

After consuming protein-rich foods, your body digests the proteins into amino acids, which are then used for muscle building and repair, among other functions. Eating protein shortly after exercising has been shown to support muscle synthesis.[101] Keep in mind that researchers disagree on the optimal amount of protein and the timing window for the best results.[102]

It's important to challenge your body—to increase the dose, intensity, speed, and frequency of your exercises and to vary them so your body can continually adapt and improve.

The Two Main Varieties of Resistance Training: Isometric and Isotonic

Isometric exercises keep joints still while the muscle group strains against the resistance. This can be done by holding planks, wall sits, and even yoga poses for two to five minutes at a time. *Isotonic* exercises involve moving muscle groups against some resistance. Examples include push-ups, sit-ups, and lifting weights. Isometric and isotonic resistance training grows muscle cells by actually damaging them first and then allowing them to recover and then repair themselves.

I highly recommend combining isometric and isotonic exercises.

There are many variations to exercise, and I am not going to get into the nitty-gritty; there are plenty of experts for that. But it's important to understand the basics. When you use muscles beyond their current capacity, which means if you go to failure or almost failure at the last repetition, the muscles respond by sustaining those microtears I mentioned. Then, during recovery, your body repairs these tears with combinations of proteins and hormones to help them grow bigger and stronger.

If your goal is to sustain health and a vibrant life, incorporate consistent resistance training workouts three times a week. You can use free weights, resistance bands, or weight machines. If you're brand-new to exercise, I recommend working with a trainer who focuses on a proper execution of movements to prevent injury.

Your Heart Is Also a Muscle

Your heart is also a muscle, and just like any other muscle, it shrinks and stiffens with physical inactivity and a sedentary lifestyle. And that can lead to an increased risk of heart disease, hypertension, and heart failure.

To have a healthy heart and lower the risk of cardiovascular diseases, it's best to exercise daily and move throughout the day. Exercise is part of a healthy life, not something we only do for a few months and expect it to last forever. Walking, easy biking, cooking, and cleaning are important aspects of daily, healthy living, not merely "exercise."

When you engage in activities like running, swimming, or cycling, your heart works harder to pump blood throughout your body, making your heart grow stronger and more efficient over time. Better blood circulation means more oxygen in all the organs and tissues, and it also helps in removing waste products from the body more efficiently. Blood pressure goes down, and mitochondrial function goes up. Healthy mitochondria in heart cells ensure that the heart has enough energy to keep pumping efficiently. Research shows that regular physical activity can lower the risk of heart disease.

Your Bones Need Muscle

Resistance training and explosive training are integral to bone health. And maintaining strong bones is essential, especially as we age. Resistance and high-impact exercises like weight lifting, jumping, and even rucking (walking with a weighted vest) are vital for building and maintaining bone density. Strong muscles support strong bones.

As we age, we need to prevent injuries and fractures. Imagine being active and traveling well into your older years without the fear of a fall. Falls can be particularly dangerous for seniors if our bones are like butter. Falls and fractures, sadly, can lead to premature death if bone health is not maintained.[103] But when you incorporate activities that stress your bones slightly, you encourage them to strengthen and build up mass, which is crucial for a healthy, active life as you get older.

Moving Is Important for Brain Health

When we exercise, the body increases the production of this incredible molecule called brain-derived neurotrophic factor (BDNF).[104] BDNF is a protein that is like a fertilizer for the brain; it is crucial for the survival, growth, and maintenance of neurons in the brain. BDNF is also vital for learning, memory, and higher thinking, and is involved in the regulation of synaptic plasticity, which is how neurons adapt in response to activity and experience.

BDNF encourages the growth and differentiation of new neurons and synapses. Synapses are the connections through which neurons communicate, and their growth is crucial for learning and memory. When we have more BDNF, we end up with improved memory, mood, and thinking, as well as lower stress, anxiety, risk of depression, and risk of Alzheimer's disease and Parkinson's disease.[105]

Exercise also stimulates the release of endorphins, which are often called the "happy hormones" because they make us feel great. These neurotransmitters produced by the central nervous system and the pituitary gland also act as natural painkillers.

The Importance of Flexibility and Balance

Balance and flexibility are crucial for optimal health because they improve physical functionality and prevent injuries. Good balance helps you maintain stability and coordination, reducing the risk of falls, especially as you age. Flexibility contributes to a greater range of motion in the joints, which aids in performing everyday activities and decreases the likelihood of muscle strains and joint stress. Better posture supported by flexibility helps optimize breathing and circulation, contributing to improved bodily functions.

Here are some ways you can improve your balance and flexibility:

- Regular stretching or yoga (even ten minutes every day at home will make a difference).
- Pilates.
- Balance exercises like standing on one leg or using a balance board (You can stand on one leg while you brush your teeth and then stand on the other while you floss).
- Dance is great for improving coordination, balance, and flexibility.
- Foam-rolling helps to release muscle tightness and improve flexibility.

Enjoy Some Time in the Sauna

The dry sauna's benefits are endless and have been studied for many years. Use of the sauna increases the expression of genes responsible for heat shock proteins (HSPs). These proteins protect cells from stress, help repair damaged proteins, scavenge free radicals, and boost glutathione production, which is the most important antioxidant produced by the liver.

The sauna also promotes muscle gains by impacting the process of muscle synthesis and breakdown. The intense heat from the sauna helps reduce protein degradation, which is important because it preserves muscle mass and function. This prevention of muscle breakdown facilitates recovery after physical exertion, enhances overall muscle health, and promotes longevity in muscle performance. Moreover, by minimizing protein degradation, the body can more efficiently repair and build muscle tissues, contributing to stronger and more resilient muscles over time.[106]

I like to use a sauna after a day of weight lifting to enhance the benefits. I do one to two rounds in one session at least three times a week, twenty minutes per one session with a cool-down break and lots of mineral water hydration before another twenty-minute session. And I admit, the sauna is also a great place to focus on thinking, reading, and relaxing.

Sauna use stimulates the production of growth hormones; it also improves insulin sensitivity, and even though you may see glucose spikes while in the sauna, this is a form of hormetic stress—a short-term stress that actually helps build resilience.[107] This process strengthens your body's ability to handle future stressors, improving both physical and mental endurance, stress management, and overall vitality.

For those who are injured and unable to work out for some time, using a sauna can be beneficial until you heal and can get back to lifting in the gym. This heat stress mimics the beneficial stress of exercise. Keep in mind that the sauna does not replace exercise; it supports your exercise plan.

Exercise Without "Exercising"

All movement is not created equally. For example, NEAT, which stands for non-exercise activity thermogenesis, refers to calories burned through all the daily activities other than formal exercise. This can be walking, gardening, cooking, and even fidgeting. The idea is to just keep moving your body or parts of your body. Other ideas include standing instead of sitting, taking the stairs instead of the elevator, and walking for short errands or while talking on the phone.

NEAT does not replace exercise. Rather, think of it as an optimal way of living daily life.

If You Must Sit, Do This

Whether you're on a long flight, driving for hours, or writing a book, it's important to move at least every forty-five minutes. Keep moving with these exercise:.

1. **Exercise snacks.** Set a timer for every forty-five to sixty minutes (this is what I do) and do any exercise you enjoy. Try short sprints, hop on an assault bike for twenty seconds and go as fast as you can, or do jumping jacks. I usually do jumping jacks, push-ups, and squats until I am out of breath. Sometimes I hop on an assault bike for twenty seconds or do battle ropes.

2. **Soleus push-ups.** This sitting move is designed to target the soleus muscle, a powerful muscle in the lower calf that plays a crucial role in walking, running, and maintaining posture. I do as many repetitions

as I can until I fatigue the muscle. Higher repetition ranges and multiple sets can be very effective.

To do soleus push-ups, the entire sole of each foot should maintain contact with the floor throughout the exercise. Begin by pressing down into the balls of your feet, trying to lift your heels off the ground. Push down through the balls of your feet to contract the soleus muscle under the load of your body weight. Hold the contraction at the top for a moment, then lower your heels back to the floor. To increase intensity, you can add weight on your knees to increase resistance. Add a dumbbell if you wish.

3. **Tabata training.** A typical Tabata protocol (developed by a Japanese doctor named Dr. Izumi Tabata) includes eight rounds of exercising for twenty seconds with high intensity, followed by ten seconds of rest. Studies show Tabata workouts can significantly improve anaerobic and aerobic fitness.[108] You can do any movement that can be done *with intensity*: fast squats, mountain climbers, high knees, walking lunges, burpees, or battle ropes.

Exercise Recovery Tips

If you are using anti-inflammatory and/or antioxidant supplements, wait a few hours to take them after your heavy lifting session. You want the acute inflammation and stress you just created with the resistance training, so you can get stronger with the adaptation. Don't blunt this with anti-inflammatory substances like vitamin C, alpha-lipoic acid, turmeric, fish oil, or other supplements. Take them at least three or more hours after working out.

My Weekly Movement Routine to Inspire You

Yoga

Each morning, I do a yoga session using an app called Glo. I vary between kundalini, flow, or Hatha yoga. My practice, which lasts between twenty to forty-five minutes, focuses on engaging my breath and mind and enhancing balance, flexibility, and strength.

Yoga positively influences gene expression by boosting energy metabolism, improving brain health, and reducing inflammatory cytokines. Cytokines are like the messengers of the immune system. They are proteins released by cells to communicate and initiate actions that help your body handle infections, inflammation, and injuries. Think of them as the emergency signals that rally the troops (other immune cells) to fight off invaders like viruses and bacteria; they also heal damaged tissue. These signals can tell the immune system to ramp up and fight hard, or sometimes, to cool down and reduce inflammation.

Gym Sessions

I lift heavy weights five times a week. But I adjust the intensity based on my menstrual cycle to prevent injuries and manage hormonal fluctuations, which is particularly important to me during perimenopause, as I am heading into menopause.

High-Intensity Interval Training

Once a week, I engage in a Norwegian 4x4 HIIT session on a bike.

Cardiovascular Activities

Each week includes a hike with a friend and three sessions of zone 2 cardiovascular training on a treadmill, during which I listen to podcasts or audiobooks.

Daily Activities

After my morning exercise, I spend most of my time standing behind my desk. I walk frequently, cook, and clean the house.

Afternoon Walk

After lunch, I put on my rucksack weighing between twenty and forty pounds, depending on my energy level, and take my dogs for a fifteen-minute uphill walk.

By maintaining steady muscle contractions throughout the day and not just during a single workout session, I ensure that my body remains active and healthy. My routine is not just about physical fitness—it keeps my brain and my mind happy and strong.

Ten Movement Ideas

Moving and exercise must be part of your life, just like brushing your teeth and getting dressed for the day. It's not an add-on; it's part of who you are and what you do. I hope these ten ideas will help you create fun daily routines.

Fall in love with daily movement. I have said it and I'll keep saying it: It's part of who we are, and it's what we are supposed to do as humans.

- Set a timer for every forty-five to sixty minutes and do ten push-ups (or as many as you can with proper form) and ten squats every time it goes off. If you start at 8:00 a.m. and end at 6:00 p.m., you will do approximately one hundred push-ups and one hundred squats per day. You will also build muscle and increase the number of push-ups and squats you can do quickly over time. Be consistent.
- Do 150 minutes a week of brisk, steady pace zone 2 exercise. Extra tip: Do a cold plunge after if you want to add more hormetic stress.
- Once a week do HIIT. Do what you enjoy the most and will consistently do—biking, rowing, battle ropes, treadmill, dance, etc. You can do the Norwegian 4x4 during this time. Rowing is great because it involves strength as well as endurance training. Supposedly rowers have the biggest heart muscles.[109]
- Park far from the grocery store entrance rather than trying to get the closest spot in order to increase movement with extra weight (groceries!). Pay attention to your posture while carrying groceries.
- Daily flexibility and balance training. This can be yoga, stretching, or Pilates. Choose what you enjoy and will do consistently.
- Once a week do explosive moves, otherwise known as plyometric exercises. They increase strength, speed, and power. Jump rope, skip around your house, slam a ball, or dance.
- Lift weights a minimum of three times each week. This should be difficult. Add a sauna session if you can for the benefits mentioned in this chapter.

- Get a standing desk, or even better, a desk treadmill for your office work.
- Walk after each meal for twenty minutes. Even dance or squats are great, as long as it's nothing too intense. This enables your body to digest food properly.
- Instead of going on restaurant dates, go on walking dates, go to playgrounds, go rock climbing, go horseback riding. You'll have more energy and have more fun!

Finally, Remember...

Exercise in itself is not the goal. Exercise is a tool to get you to the goal, which is to feel, function, and look great for all or most of your life. Also, be sure you eat enough clean protein and cultivate a healthy digestive system to break down protein into amino acids to be used to build your strong body.

CHAPTER FIVE

YOUR INNER ENVIRONMENT

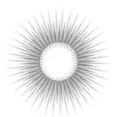

In the spring of 2022, I faced significant gastrointestinal (GI) issues that kept me confined to my home for several weeks. I was scared. After undergoing tests, I discovered my pancreas was barely producing enzymes. The fear of facing a serious health condition was overwhelming, especially with the thought of pancreatic complications.

At that time, my greatest desire was to be present for my daughter, Summer, who was two years away from graduating from high school. My thoughts were consumed with the time I hoped to spend with her.

I soon realized that the root of my GI problems was tied to my emotional childhood trauma, particularly connected to my mother. I dedicated two months to intense emotional work, confronting and processing the traumas of my childhood. Slowly, I noticed my health starting to improve.

All I wanted was to be there for Summer as she embarked on her adult life. The love for my daughter and the strong desire to enjoy my life pulled me toward healing.

For a long time, I struggled to accept that I was a victim of abuse. I normalized my pain. Despite years of therapy and hypnosis aimed at healing my trauma, I never allowed myself to truly feel sorry for my experiences. I always thought everyone had a painful story, and mine was no different. I have always focused on learning lessons from adversity. I was working on healing and breaking the family cycle to be free and feel happy, yet there was something I needed to dig deeper into.

My relationship with my mother has always been complicated, especially since my father's death in 2014. Her unresolved anger toward him, and subsequently toward me as I resisted her manipulations, weighed heavily on me. Growing up amid constant violence and abuse, isolation became normal. In such an environment where therapy was scarce, voicing my troubles seemed unjustified. I was often reminded by my mother of how hard my parents' lives were and how mine was "good enough." I believed it was my role to absorb the pains of emotional and physical abuse silently.

One morning in April 2022, during meditation, I started receiving messages, images, and feelings about my mother and my childhood pain. I grabbed a pen and my journal and started to write everything down.

My body was sending clear signals that it was time for a change. That month, my physical symptoms became unbearable. Night after night, I was awakened by severe discomfort in my intestines, so intense I couldn't sleep. I was scared; I did not know what was happening.

Thankfully, I knew the only way to discover the source of my pain and discomfort was to run lab tests. Medical tests revealed significantly low pancreatic enzymes, dropping two hundred points from my last regular stool test. The symptoms kept getting worse every day.

I started to read and learn more about pancreatitis and pancreatic cancer. I did not want to die yet. I had to pull myself together and start emotional trauma work. It was time to release my mother; it was time to cut the cord. My body was crying out, wanting to release it all.

I called my doctor to get an ultrasound of my organs. No tumor! I was relieved. I needed to rule out all physical possibilities of any kind of disease.

I realized that these physical manifestations were directly tied to the emotional traumas I had carried unknowingly for years. It wasn't about the food I ate or my lifestyle habits; it was about the toxic inner environment I had nurtured. I had been unaware of how I normalized the experiences from my childhood, until encouragement from a friend changed things for me.

During my regular acupuncture session, a simple, compassionate, loving hand from my practitioner and dear friend, Oona, allowed me to finally confront my pain. As she looked at me and said, "What happened to you sucks, and it's okay to feel sorry for yourself," her validation unleashed all that I had normalized, all that was stuck inside my body, marking the beginning of my true healing process.

That night after this session, I had a clear dream. It was a message from my higher self, telling me to see Oona, my acupuncturist, every single day for two weeks to heal. I messaged her that morning to let her know that I needed her. Learning to ask for help had taken many years, but I knew this was also part of my journey. She was happy to help me.

Each session brought me into a state of deep relaxation and dreams. I connected to my inner source, cried with joy, and wasn't afraid anymore. I trusted my body and was grateful to be surrounded by people who loved and cared about me. My higher self guided me through the next few weeks.

I had daily acupuncture sessions and dedicated time in my room, embracing practices of deep internal healing. I journaled, meditated, and allowed myself to grieve and heal, gradually peeling away the layers of trauma, working on cutting the cord and forgiving my mother for her abuse.

This experience taught me a vital lesson: Our physical health reflects our emotional chronic stress from past experiences, especially childhood. By addressing and healing our inner traumas, we can transform our entire well-being.

True health is understanding and nurturing the complex interplay between our minds, bodies, and spirits. Embrace the journey, and trust that with the right support and inner work, transformation is possible!

Awareness Is the First Step

Sometimes we do not know why we feel anxious in certain situations. We don't know why we react to certain people, words, or places in a way we don't like. Why are we shy or outgoing? Why do we like being alone? Why do we always need company to feel safe? Why do we have all these thoughts on repeat about ourselves—blame, shame, guilt?

The only way to know is to become still, to do practices that will bring us closer to our inner self so we can become aware of who we truly are deep down.

There is an incredible wisdom deep within all of us that wants to talk to us, wants to come through, if we just stop and become still every day, even for just a few minutes. If we pay attention, let all the stored pain, disappointments, and traumas come to the surface, we can live a happier and healthier life. It is not always comfortable, but it's worth it, because on the other side is peace, freedom, and true health.

I encourage you to take a moment to sit quietly, feel, and write. Simply let your thoughts flow as you sit in stillness. Even if you believe there's nothing new to discover, or that your health issues aren't connected to your past or emotions, it's important to do this work. If you truly want to achieve the health you dream of, this reflection is essential.

You may be able to completely change your relationship with health, food, exercise, and sleep. It does not need to be a huge traumatic event. Trauma may be from a time when someone made a comment about your weight, or the way you eat, and that left a scar inside.

Perhaps you have certain habits that don't serve you, and you just can't figure out why you can't let them go. Whatever it is, if you keep ignoring these issues and hope they will disappear, they will keep growing inside of your body like tumors. Suppressed emotions will manifest physically, leading to symptoms like back pain or digestive issues.

Imagine who you would be without the stories, the pains, the stuff that happened to you after you've released them. Just imagine it! What is keeping you from becoming fully aware, connecting you to your emotions?

Many of us are waiting for the perfect moment to address the challenges we have, but this perfect moment never arrives because life is always in motion.

Why wait for your health to decline when you can take proactive steps now?

External circumstances may not change; it's up to us to find our own rhythm and balance, to know when to say no, when to unwind, and when to make necessary changes to alleviate stress.

The body doesn't distinguish between actual experiences and thoughts. You can literally alter your biology, chemistry, hormones, and genes through the power of your inner dialogue.[110] By changing the narratives we tell ourselves, we can transform our physical and mental states.

Stop Letting Trauma Control Your Health—and Your Destiny

What if unresolved trauma is the cause of all or most of your health challenges, from bloating to headaches to cancer? We don't realize how deeply affected we are by traumatic events that happen to most of us, especially in childhood when we are most vulnerable and dependent.

We need to start talking about trauma openly. People who were victimized are told that they're not supposed to feel shame and guilt. We need to feel comfortable talking about our traumas to release them! This was one of my big lessons, and I can guarantee you, it will change your life for the better if you do this deep, uncomfortable work.

What is the most traumatic experience you have had? Do you even remember it? What hurts you? Is it the loss of someone you loved and haven't allowed yourself to grieve? Is it being abandoned or made fun of?

Maybe you had poor sleep or eating routines when you were a child, and that is stressful now too. What is your relationship with food and exercise? How are you sleeping? I encourage you to answer these questions and ask yourself why your relationship to food or exercise is what it is. The answers are shaped by our experiences in childhood and young adulthood. Trauma changes us on a cellular level; it changes how our genes are expressed. And that's why you must invite the traumas to come out of your body with compassion and love instead of shame and guilt. The trauma is not your fault; you have nothing to be ashamed of. Only when we acknowledge the behavior that is not serving us can the healing begin. Do not normalize the pain you have experienced.

If you've experienced trauma, you likely have behaviors that are getting in the way of you being able to achieve optimal health. I urge you to be curious, to wonder where the pain may be coming from. Pay attention to everyday triggers; they may be connecting to deep, unresolved wounds. There is so much freedom in knowing. Although it takes hard work to heal, it's much harder to live with uncovered trauma for the rest of your life. Your health is worth the work!

Feel sad, be angry, and feel disappointment. Feel all the emotions that come through you. Sit with the emotions so they can be processed and released. If this is a foreign subject for you, hire a life coach or therapist you trust who can help you go deep, help you feel, and help you release.

Explore Your Inner Environment

Everything we do, think, and feel, as well as the people that are in our lives, affects our inner environment—including the food we eat, the exercises we do, and how we sleep.

Our *inner environment* refers to all the thoughts, emotions, beliefs, self-created stories, and experiences that affect our overall mental and physical state. The inner environment is the internal landscape that influences how we see and interact with the world around us.

One reason I love practicing kundalini yoga and pran-ayama breathing techniques is because of how they alter my inner environment in a very short time. I also get a similar experience from doing a cold plunge.

If you focus and believe in healing, you increase the body's ability to heal. If you believe in the person you want to become, you are more likely to become it. If you believe and focus on what you desire instead of what you resist, you are more likely to achieve your desired health. It's not only food and exercise, but also your thoughts that regulate your hormones, which then regulate your mood. As uncomfort-able as it may be for many, plunging my body into cold water is the fastest way to make myself feel invigorated and joyful.

The connection between our thoughts and physiolog-ical responses is complex but well-supported by scientific research. Our beliefs and our thoughts create emotions. These emotions are regulated by hormones. If you have positive thoughts, which can take place during meditation or visual-ization, your body will release hormones like serotonin. This hormone makes you feel calm and joyful. You also release endorphins, the natural painkillers that improve mood and brain health.

On the other hand, by merely imagining a stressful situation, your body will produce cortisol, the stress hormone, which will then create reactions in the body that promote inflammation. While acute stress can sometimes be beneficial, chronic, ongoing stress that we may not even be aware of can silently causing your health issues.

When you explore your inner environment, you get in touch with your true self, which allows you to truly heal and thrive in all aspects of life.

Transform Your Identity

Shift your mindset, shift your health.

This principle guides my work, and I see its truth unfold daily in the lives of many people.

If you've ever struggled with believing you don't deserve love or joy, or felt doomed by persistent health issues like headaches, poor gut health, and extra weight, know that these are common stories.

I'm often moved by stories from my clients who suffer silently, believing that chronic discomfort is part of life. Many come to me after years of suffering, having been down the traditional routes of medication without success. They're desperate for change but skeptical that anything different can happen. I understand.

My friend, a deep thinker and empath, asked me to look into the high sensitivity trait. I believed I was too sensitive and thinking too much and too deeply about life and experiences. I felt that people couldn't understand me. I believed something was wrong with me. My horrific self-talk was making me miserable and affecting my physical health.

My daughter, Summer, and I are both highly sensitive people (HSPs). Being aware of and understanding this trait, though challenging, has transformed our lives for the better once we understood it. It's not just about sensitivity; it's the ability to process deeply and so much more. We had to learn about harnessing this trait to foster a deeper connection with our health.

Knowing this allowed me to change my identity. I am an HSP; I am not crazy, too intuitive, too sensitive, too much... I changed my self-talk completely to self-talk that serves my emotional and physical health. I encourage you to explore Dr. Elaine Aron's work about HSPs, perhaps starting with the documentary we were part of, *Sensitive: The Untold Story* (sensitivethemovie.com).

If you are an HSP, knowing and understanding this trait will change your life for the better. Your identity shapes how you see yourself and how you interact with the world. It's often a story we tell ourselves based on past experiences. Negative self-talk, such as, *I am always sick, I am fat,* or *No one cares about me,* are merely stories we've told ourselves for so long that we end up becoming those people.

But what if you could rewrite that narrative? Imagine replacing those thoughts with: *I am lovable, My life is filled with joy,* or *I am healthy and strong.* What if? What do you have to lose? You can only gain from changing the narrative with daily practice.

Just as a forest doesn't recover overnight from a fire, changing ingrained beliefs takes time and effort. It starts with challenging the truth of your negative stories. Inspired by Byron Katie's book *Loving What Is,* I encourage you to question your beliefs.[111] Are the negative thoughts you believe about yourself and your health genuinely true? Most often they are not.

Visualize who you want to be a year from now. What habits, what kind of health, what kind of relationships do you see? Create that vision and start living it now. This isn't about positive thinking; it's about creating who you desire to be, a new identity, and a new you!

The internal family systems (IFS) model can be a powerful tool as well. It's a form of psychotherapy developed by Dr. Richard C. Schwartz in the 1980s. IFS is based on the idea that our mind is naturally subdivided into a number of different parts or subpersonalities, each with its own perspective, feelings, and role. IFS is used to treat a variety of psychological issues, including trauma, anxiety, depression, and eating disorders. IFS emphasizes self-compassion and understanding. It helps us understand the various parts of our personality, why they exist, and how to work with them. IFS is an extremely helpful tool for achieving inner freedom and peace.[112]

It's time to drop the old stories that no longer serve you. As you step into this new identity, practice it daily. When old thoughts sneak up on you, gently acknowledge them and let them go. Remind yourself, *That's not me anymore.*

There are many ways to care for our inner environment. At the end of this chapter, I will list the ones I have used during my own healing journey and continue to use. I suggest you choose one at a time so you don't get overwhelmed and can experience it enough so that it makes an impact.

All the modalities and tools I've used have impacted my life and continue to do so. They will also bring you something unique. Listen to your feelings as you go through the list, and let your intuition guide you toward what may be the most important book, meditation, or practice to use right now in your process.

But whatever you choose, the key is to show up every day for yourself with an open heart. Listen to your inner guidance, and you will find your way to health and healing. Consistency is key to success.

Connect Your Purpose

I always believed my purpose was to be happy. In fact, I believed *everyone's* purpose was to be happy.

However, it dawned on me at some point that the true purpose of life is to live in your truth, to be who you are in the core of yourself, to heal from pains, and to enjoy what appear to be the small gifts of life yet are the biggest, like the morning sun and the butterflies flying around the blooming flowers.

Pause and feel your body. Focus on what provides a feeling of peace, freedom, and contentment—the feeling of being lost in time, where you enjoy what you are doing, when you are feeling energized and filled with love.

Is there something you do that makes you feel fulfilled and content? It can be making art, playing music, riding a bike, learning about the human brain, cooking, math, building with LEGOs, talking to people...any activity that inspires you, really.

What is it? Don't just move on and keep reading. Pause and feel it. What is it for you that fills your heart?

Whatever that is, your purpose is what makes you feel aligned, what gives you the true feeling of happiness inside. I believe we all have "it" and know it deep down, yet we can't get there until we give ourselves the chance to listen to and trust ourselves.

I have always felt happy taking care of others, teaching and guiding people, and seeing their health turn around and shine with joy, seeing how capable they are and how much better they feel. I want the same results for you.

This is where I am truly myself. I have been like this since I was a child, and that is why I do the work I do; it's what fulfills me the most.

How I Maintain a Healthy Inner Environment

I've always had a busy mind. The idea of shutting it off to focus on stillness, even for just three minutes, used to seem impossible. I am a thinker, and I used to believe that meditation was too difficult despite knowing how beneficial it could be for my nervous system and connecting with my intuition.

Yet something inside me said to keep showing up every morning and reading about meditation. So I persisted, showing up every morning in the same little room of our rented house back in 2013. Over time, this routine became more than just a practice; it became a part of my identity. I don't even call it meditation, even after all these years. I refer to it as my morning practice.

Each session is different, but some elements are consistent. For example, every morning I wake up between 5:00 and 5:30 a.m., and lie in bed with my eyes closed, lingering in the alpha state as I review my dreams, feelings, and inner voice with curiosity. After a few minutes reflecting on my night, I say thank-you for the new, great day ahead. Then I get up, go to the bathroom, scrape my tongue, and head to the kitchen to drink two large glasses of filtered water while gazing out at the sky, setting an intention for my day.

Then I move to my Zen room. Depending on what I feel guided to do that morning, I may journal or simply sit with my eyes closed, listening to binaural beats or a guided meditation. I do a quick breathwork session and read inspirational words. I don't plan this; I follow my intuition for what I need each morning. This is followed by a short yoga practice. Around 7:00 a.m., I'm ready to go to the gym.

This morning practice is who I am and what I do, and I have no plans to change it, because it serves me well. This practice supports my emotional, physical, and spiritual health.

This routine is how I show myself self-love and take care of my inner environment. Of course, some people believe that routine can make us dull. But I believe we do better as humans when we have *some* routines. Our brains and bodies thrive in routines because they create a sense of stability and predictability, reducing stress and anxiety. Consistent habits allow us to conserve energy by automating daily tasks, freeing up mental resources for creativity and problem-solving.

How to Nurture Your Inner Environment

Begin each new day with clear intentions. Decide what kind of day you want to have, giving yourself the chance to live the life you truly desire. Remember, every thought you think can be changed. Thoughts lead to feelings, which lead to actions. By choosing different thoughts, you can change how you feel, which will change your actions.

Consider these two simple questions each morning to nurture your inner environment:

- How do I feel right now?
- How do I want to feel today?

Your mind is a powerful tool, and you can retrain it to think in ways that truly serve you. Believe in your inner wisdom and intelligence. You have the power to make life as challenging or as rewarding as you believe it can be. I know all these suggestions may be difficult for many, but they are simple to do, and take only a little bit of time in your day. They work. I know they do, because they have transformed my life and the lives of many others.

Nurture Yourself in Nature

Things outside of yourself can make dramatic changes to how you feel. And here I mean literally outside—stepping into nature to touch a tree or walk barefoot on grass. Activities like this will energize your body and restore your spirit.

Go to a park, forest, lake, or the beach. Lie down on the ground to literally ground yourself and calm your nervous system down. If you live in a city with no close proximity to nature, get resourceful. Buy as many plants as you possibly can take care of for your home. Create a natural environment inside your home.

Step out of your front door and look up into the sky in wonder. Listen to the birds, the air moving, the wind. Sit and observe. Do nothing. Talk to no one. Read nothing. Just be.

Practice this daily for at least five minutes. Slowly but surely, you will notice positive shifts in your inner environment. I promise!

Laughter Really Is the Best Medicine

Laughing not only boosts your immune system and lowers your blood pressure, but it also stimulates the release of endorphins while reducing cortisol levels.[113] But beyond the science, laughing just feels so darn good! Laugh as much as possible.

Clarify and Heal Through the Power of Writing

It's fascinating how the act of writing allows us to come to terms with trauma and other negative emotions. By expressing yourself to yourself, you can let go of the toxic thoughts. And the more you write, the more clarity you will gain, and the better you will feel about the past, present, and future.

There are no rules for journaling. All you need is a pen and paper. There are no limitations. It doesn't matter if you have messy penmanship; it doesn't matter if what you write makes no sense at all. The power of journaling comes from the literal act of putting the words and sentences on the page.

Write anytime about anything, whatever comes to mind: the breakfast you made in the morning, a work colleague who has been annoying you, the puppy you had as a five-year-old, an abusive relationship, whatever. Write about happy memories too. It's about getting it all out and letting it go.

We don't want to ruminate or suppress our emotions. Avoiding your feelings or running away from them isn't just impossible, it makes everything harder to address later on. Journaling is the tool that eliminates the feelings and thoughts that aren't serving you, providing a stairway into a blissful future.

But you have to be honest with yourself and let the thoughts flow freely without editing yourself. Don't hesitate to confront your shortcomings and mistakes. What lessons can you learn from them? How can they be appreciated?

Journaling is like emptying the cup of your mind and heart. By confronting and acknowledging your past, it stops it from shaping your future; the past trauma is being released from your organs, and from the subconscious mind. So sit down and start writing.

Meditation

Getting into the body and asking the mind to let go may be a difficult task for many of us, and yet when we do this practice daily, it is profound, freeing, so beautiful, and so worth our time. Meditation is the a simple practice of becoming more you. It is one of the most beneficial activities for developing a strong inner environment. That's because meditation is the practice of awareness, of being present, of being here now. And only when you're aware can you truly get in touch with the issues preventing you from flourishing in the world.

Meditation allows me to get to know my true inner self. Doing so allows me to manage daily stressors and accept things I can't control with more ease. I know myself more. I can notice the rise of those uncomfortable feelings before they take over my mind. Well, it's a work in progress: I notice them some of the time, and my goal is to notice them most of the time. The point is, showing up daily for my morning practice has made me a much better person to myself and to those around me. The same can happen for you.

When you sit in meditation, the goal isn't to force specific feelings or thoughts. You might use tools like breath to calm your nervous system or focus on a neutral sound, but you don't need anything. Simply being in the moment is powerful enough.

This practice of being in the moment will signal to your cells that you are safe and will be deeply healing to your body. You can observe your breath and let your thoughts come and go without analyzing them. Just let them pass by.

I have heard meditation teachers use this analogy: Think of your thoughts as clouds floating by in the sky; watch them drift away until you find yourself in a state of calm stillness.

As you sit quietly, your breath will slow, and you might find a smile spreading across your face or tears rolling down your cheeks. This happens to me sometimes. Whatever emotions arise, allow them to go where they may; it's all part of the process. Keep a notebook and pen next to you to reflect and release what's needed.

Whatever comes is meant to come. Embrace it.

Here are some different approaches to meditation. Explore them all to see what resonates with your soul.

Mantra Meditation

A mantra is a word, sound, or phrase that you repeat to help with concentration in meditation. It originates from ancient Sanskrit, where *man* means "mind" and *tra* means "tool" or "instrument." Therefore, a mantra is a tool for the mind. Repeating a phrase or a word calms the mind and soul. It should be something that feels good to you. Examples: *I am at peace. I am safe. I am worthy. I am loved.*

Body-Scan Meditation

Scan your body by putting your intention on each part of the body as you go from top to bottom or from the soles of your feet to the crown of your head. This focused meditation, also called *yoga nidra*, is very calming on the nervous system and keeps you focused on your body instead of your thoughts.

I like doing this particular practice in bed before I go to sleep, though some of my clients enjoy doing their own body scan as part of their morning routine. No matter when you do it, it keeps your mind focused on your body, and you feel calmer and more grounded.

Hypnosis

Hypnosis is a state of focused mind where the mind is highly responsive to suggestions. Did you know that when you are watching TV, you are in a hypnotic state? This is because you are deeply focused and absorbed, similar to the focused state induced during hypnosis.[114] Hypnosis is a great way to heal the mind and soul. During hypnosis, the conscious mind takes a break, allowing the subconscious mind to become more accessible. This state makes it easier to accept positive suggestions and make changes in thoughts, feelings, and behaviors. You can do hypnosis with a practitioner, or try one of the apps available for self-hypnosis.

Music

In a poll conducted by the University of Michigan of 2,500 adults between fifty and eighty years old, 98 percent felt at least one benefit from engaging with music, 41 percent said that music is vital to their well-being, and 60 to 75 percent reported that music gave them more energy, motivation, less stress, better mood, relaxation, and joy.[115]

Whether listening to music, playing an instrument, or singing in a choir, music had a meaningful impact on the cohort's overall health and well-being, providing far more

than just entertainment. An incredible 31 percent of partici-
pants reported that music helps keep their mind sharp, and
7 percent reported ease of pain while listening to music.[116]
Music has benefits for everything from lowering blood pressure to easing depression.

Breathing Practices

1. **Double inhale:** Long exhales calm the nervous
   system quickly. Take one long inhale and another
   short inhale right after, then a long, slow exhale. Do
   this three times for a quick physiological change to
   your nervous system.
2. **Box breathing:** Breathe in for four seconds, hold for
   four, breathe out for four, hold for four. Repeat until
   you feel calm. Change the number of seconds so it's
   comfortable for you. Do not force anything.
3. The **4-7-8 breath** is a simple breathing technique
   designed to promote relaxation and reduce stress.
   Here's how it works: Inhale quietly through your
   nose for a count of four. Hold your breath for a count
   of seven. Exhale completely through your mouth,
   making a *whoosh* sound, for a count of eight. This
   cycle is considered one breath. Repeat as needed to
   help calm your mind and body.
4. Drop your tongue to the bottom of your mouth and
   relax your jaw. Close your eyes, breathe, and just be.

Connect to Your Body

Since the body and mind are so intertwined, here are a
few more practices to calm your mind by connecting with
your body:

Feel Your Pulse

If you feel stressed, place the thumb of one hand on the other hand's wrist and connect to your pulse. If your pulse feels rapid and strong, it may indicate that your body is in a heightened state of stress. To counteract this, use any of the breathing tools mentioned earlier. By consciously breathing and tuning in to your pulse, you can help shift your body from a state of stress to one of calm.

Head Hold

Place one hand on your head, the other on your belly. Close your eyes and breathe. This grounding, simple moment will feel like a warm hug.

Heart Hold

Place one hand on your heart and the other on your belly. Close your eyes and breathe to feel calmness.

Eye Hold

Rub your hands together to create heat. Place them over your eyes but not touching your eyelids, then close your eyes and feel the warm, calming ease that comes with this practice.

Emotional Freedom Technique

The Emotional Freedom Technique (EFT) is a tapping practice that involves tapping on specific acupressure points on the body while focusing on and verbalizing the issue or emotion that is triggering you and creating fear, worry, or anger.[117] This helps to address and neutralize the emotional response, allowing you to settle into a state of safety and calm. This technique is often used to alleviate stress, anxiety, phobias, and other emotional challenges.

Yoga

Yoga combines movement with breath, creating a powerful practice that can calm the nervous system. Engaging in yoga, even for just five minutes, can help reset and soothe your nervous system. Yoga emphasizes deep, controlled breathing, which activates the parasympathetic nervous system. This promotes relaxation. The deliberate and slow movements in yoga help shift focus away from stressors and into the body and the present moment, also promoting relaxation.

Panoramic Vision

Panoramic vision is a technique that helps reduce stress and promote relaxation. To practice it, keep your head and body steady, and look out at the sky or far away into nature. Move your eyes to scan gently from side to side. This practice engages your peripheral vision, which can help activate the parasympathetic nervous system, leading to a state of calm and relief.[118] Incorporating panoramic vision into your daily routine can be a simple yet powerful way to manage stress and improve your overall sense of well-being.

Cold Therapy

If you are overthinking, stressed, sluggish, depressed, or anxious, try a cold plunge, cold shower, or even ice cubes on your face and hands. Just be careful if you have any health conditions like high blood pressure or a viral infection that may make this fun activity unsafe for you.

The benefits:
- Your mind stops all the thinking—it really stops!
- Your mood is regulated thanks to the release of adrenaline.
- You get an energy boost.
- This decreases the chance of infection from viruses and bacteria by lowering inflammation in the body.[119]

Ask for Help

No one is meant to do everything on their own. We need community. We do better with loving support from others. We can only do so much on our own. This is why we need to ask others for help.

I know it's hard to do—I used to be there! I believed I had to suffer alone in silence. I had to learn as an adult to ask for help. That took years, but once I started to give people a chance to help me, I realized how important it is to seek a helping hand and heart.

Remember: There is always someone out there ready to help!

How are you feeling? I know it's a lot to process. I have been sharing many tools and practices I have discovered and found to be helpful over the years. I invite you to pause for a moment and decide which one step, which one practice, you need the most right now, and simply do that. Remember, taking one small step consistently will have a much bigger impact in the long term than trying to adopt too many new practices and habits all at once.

My Favorite Healing Resources

These are some of the modalities, practices, books, and therapies I have used on my journey of healing. While the journey never stops, it does gets easier and easier.

I continue to use many of these resources, and they have been enjoyed by my friends, family members, and clients:

- Books and meditations by author Gabby Bernstein
- EFT, Emotional Freedom Technique
- Books and meditations by Joe Dispenza, who provides powerful, science-based ways to change your identity and to heal
- The book *You Can Heal Your Life* by Louise Hay (Hay House, 1984)
- Events and books by Tony Robbins
- IFS, internal family system therapy
- The book *The Seat of the Soul* and corresponding program by Gary Zukav (Simon and Schuster, 2014)
- Somatic work (focuses on how emotions and experiences are stored in the body)
- Acupuncture
- Massage to relax and ground
- Kundalini yoga and breathing practices
- The breathwork method of Wim Hof
- Cold plunge
- The book *Stillness Is the Key* by Ryan Holiday (Portfolio, 2019)
- Books by Ram Dass
- Self-hypnosis apps such as Reveri, Harmony, or HypnoBox

- The book *The Biology of Belief: Unleashing the Power of Consciousness, Matter, and Miracles* by Bruce H. Lipton (Hay House, 2010)
- The book *Trauma: The Invisible Epidemic* by Paul Conti (Vermilion, 2022)
- Apps for meditation, breathing techniques, and more:
  - Insight Timer: music, meditation, yoga, and more
  - Glo: yoga and meditation
  - Breethe: hypnosis
  - iBreathe: breathwork
  - Binaural: app for specific binaural sounds (great tool for meditations—I listen to alpha or theta waves during meditation)
  - Brain.fm: music
  - HeartMath: app and device to monitor and improve your heart rate variability, enhancing emotional regulation

Our mental and emotional state strongly affects our physical health and shapes how we experience the world. By understanding and embracing the deep connection between your mind and body, you can transform the way you feel, think, and live. Cultivating mindfulness, self-awareness, and going deep, doing the emotional work that you need to do, is about supporting your overall health.

When you are taking care of your inner environment, your life is better, and you gain the power to thrive in every aspect of your life. Listen to your body, nurture your mind, and empower yourself with these tools to create lasting, vibrant health from the inside out.

CHAPTER SIX

TRANSFORMATION: HOW TO CREATE THE CHANGE YOU DEEPLY DESIRE

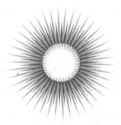

When my clients are in the process of transforming their identity and ask how I manage to eat out with friends who indulge in alcohol and fried foods, I share a simple truth with them about my identity: I am someone who doesn't drink alcohol or eat fried food.

Now, giving up alcohol was a breeze for me, but fried foods? That was a tough one. You see, I grew up in Slovakia on fried meat and cheese—it was a staple at home and at family gatherings. And let's be honest, fried food is everywhere. But I value my health. I know too well the harmful effects fried foods can have on the body, particularly inflammation and oxidative stress, which can impact gut and brain function. That understanding was my turning point. I made a conscious decision to eliminate fried foods from my diet entirely. I told everyone around me as a way of holding myself accountable and so everyone would understand that this is a nonnegotiable for me.

To make it easier, I used to joke that I picture fried foods as cigarette butts. Sounds unappealing, right? I'd ask myself, "Why would you ever eat cigarette butts?" That worked for me, and I no longer even desired fried foods. It became part of who I am. This change wasn't just about avoiding certain foods; it was about redefining how I see myself and making choices that align with the healthiest version of me.

In this chapter, we'll dive deep into creating your own strategies for lasting change. You'll learn how to incorporate small, healthy actions into your daily routine that gradually become second nature. While motivation is necessary, we can't rely on it. Strategy provides results.

Create a New Identity

As described in the previous chapter, identity is defining who you are. Your identity is the foundation of your being; it shapes your perceptions, the stories you hold on to, your behaviors, your habits, and how you live in this world.

Your identity is how you perceive yourself in the present moment, how you think of yourself, how you describe yourself. And those beliefs can hinder you from walking the path you envision for yourself. It's important to be truly aware of who you are at this moment. What are your values, beliefs, strengths, challenges, and characteristics? Do you hear yourself describing yourself as any of these?

- I am not a good sleeper.
- I have always been fat.
- I am not good at focusing on one thing; I have always been like this.
- I have always had migraines and there is nothing I can do about it.
- I can't meditate.
- I am anxious.
- I don't like to exercise.
- This is just who I am (sad face).

You get the point, right?

Whatever beliefs you are holding on to, if they are not serving you, it's time to let them go and create a new you. You can decide to change your identity in one minute. I'm serious. You can decide right now: *I am a person who walks every morning. I love eating vegetables for breakfast. I fall asleep with ease every night. I enjoy writing in my journal every morning. I am healthy. I am free of ... I can do ... I am able to ... I want to ... I am ...* Fill in the blank.

I am not suggesting that you can lie to yourself and instantly become this new version of yourself. I am saying that you can choose your thoughts right now. The thoughts that play in your mind on repeat will determine your feelings and your behaviors every day of your life, creating your life.

Before you can create a new identity, you must spend time with yourself and know yourself; you must feel safe to see yourself truly for who you are right now. This step is crucial and can't be skipped. Get your rails down, be vulnerable, go deep, let your brain go, and feel into your truth. Try more of the practices from the previous chapter to get there.

Understanding your current identity helps you gain clarity on your values, strengths, passions, and areas for improvement. This self-awareness is crucial for setting meaningful goals. Goals set without this foundational understanding might lack authenticity and alignment with your true self, leading to less consistent motivation and eventually fulfillment.

As you go through this process of creating the person you deeply desire to become, know there will be people who may not be supportive and happy about these changes.

One of the most significant lessons I've learned is the power of standing in your truth. For me, this meant leaving behind everything familiar to pursue a life aligned with my deepest values and beliefs. Despite being raised in an environment of turmoil and suppression, I chose to stand up for what I believed in, even when it meant facing rejection or misunderstanding, criticism, and judgment from my parents and other family members. Do not settle out of fear; you will attract the right people as you start the shift. I know it's not easy, trust me. I have done it, and many others have, so you can too! You'll be glad you did.

You will surely experience fear and self-doubt if you break away from your normal pack. Every human does; it's natural. When those feelings arise, focus on your *why*—the deep-seated reasons driving your transformation. The *why* is what pulls you—it is the light to focus on; it's what helps you overcome all obstacles.

Practical Exercise: Changing Your Identity

Before moving on to creating a vision for your new life, take some time to reflect on and redefine who you are. Here are two simple questions to guide you through this process:

1. What are your current values, beliefs, and strengths? Reflect on what you currently believe about yourself and your life that is serving you well.

2. What are your current unwanted beliefs and challenges? Identify which beliefs are no longer serving you.

Create Your Vision

Just as you set a destination in your GPS to know how to get to your destination, a health and life vision is a clear direction and goal for your future; it helps you define what you desire to achieve and where you want to go.

Your vision serves as a constant reminder, helping you stay on track just like the GPS helps you stay on the route you chose. Vision helps you prioritize what is important to you.

While creating your vision, don't pressure yourself with a strict timeline. In some cases, a timeline is important; it helps provide structure and motivation. For others, it might lead to stress. I do not like to use too many rules here. Again, listen to your inner voice, the truth inside you. As you use my simple guide below, adjust it to how it best works for you. Your vision might shift as circumstances change, so be flexible. Reflect and reevaluate as you keep going.

Whatever you do, whatever your pace, creating a vision for the future helps align your daily actions with your long-term aspirations. Here's how to get started:

Set the Scene

The ideal time to create vision is in the morning, as the sun rises. It's quiet and peaceful, before the rush of the day takes over. Go to a cozy space where you will not be interrupted. Get a pen and paper and go through the questions I offer below. Be clear, specific, and descriptive in your desires.

A study found that you become 42 percent more likely to achieve your goals and dreams simply by writing them down regularly.[120]

Define What You Desire

First, let's explore desire. Desire is a feeling that pulls you toward your goals. You want something new in your life: more energy, greater physical strength, healthier skin, increased focus, improved memory.

- **If you were granted three wishes right now, with no cost, no effort, what would those be?** Just write them down now. If you have a desire, it means it is already a possibility, since you have already envisioned it in your mind.

We are energetic beings. If you can have a thought and imagine yourself being, doing, and feeling something—anything—then that is what you are creating. Get as clear and specific as you can. See it. Feel it. Be it. Anything you desire is possible if you believe it. Go big! Your answers to these questions will help describe your future life and why you want it. Your health and life matter. Write all your answers in positive language: "I will" rather than "I won't." For example: "I will be in bed by 10 p.m." or "I will walk after each meal."

To help you get a clearer picture of the person you want to become, ask yourself these guiding questions:

- **What does my daily routine look like?** Think about your day from start to finish. For example, do you begin your day with meditation or exercise, or do you jump straight into work? What do your habits look like throughout the day? What is your bedtime routine?
- **What foods am I eating?** Picture the meals that nourish both your body and mind. Are you fueling your body with nutritious, real, whole foods or relying on processed, quick-fix meals?
- **What am I doing for fun?** How do you unwind? It could be as simple as a walk in nature, reading a good book, or dancing to your favorite music.
- **What is my relationship with myself?** Are you kind and compassionate toward yourself? Do you practice self-care and speak to yourself with love and encouragement?
- **How do I want to be thinking every day?** You might want your thoughts to be positive, clear, and focused on gratitude and possibilities. For example, instead of dwelling on problems, you could shift your mindset to focus on solutions and things you're thankful for. In that case, you could answer: *I want to be thinking positively, with a clear mind and focused on gratitude and possibilities.*
- **What do I want to be feeling every day?** Consider how you want to feel. Do you want to wake up feeling energetic, vibrant, and ready to take on the day? Imagine moving through your life feeling light, joyful, and full of purpose.

Now that you've identified where you are and what you want, the following questions answer the *why* for your desires. These questions will help you understand the deeper reasons behind your goals:

- **What am I able *to do* when I am this person, feeling and thinking this way?** Example answer: *When I feel energetic and think positively, I can exercise regularly, engage in activities I love, and tackle daily tasks with more ease.*
- **What am I able *to have* when I am this person, feeling and thinking this way?** Example answer: *I can have a balanced, fulfilling life with strong relationships and excellent physical health.*
- **How will these changes within me *benefit other people*?** Example answer: *These changes will allow me to be more present and supportive for my family and friends, inspiring them to have better health.*

Believe and Expect

French hypnotist Emile Coué said, "If you induce in yourself a belief that you can do a certain thing, you are going to do it, no matter how difficult it may be."

Our minds are incredibly powerful tools that can influence our reality. Think about the power of the placebo effect—this is when beliefs cause actual changes in our bodies. The placebo effect demonstrates our ability to influence our health through mindset. Just the same, limiting beliefs will block you from manifesting desires.

It is not what you want that you create; you create what you believe to be true. Belief is confidence in the outcome. Have fun with it. If you believe something, go after it!

Add Gratitude

Now, write your new identity based on your desires with gratitude.

Take your answers to the questions above and write a clear and concise vision statement including the *whys* that encapsulate your long-term goals and desired future, as if you're already there. You are grateful for your new life, your new identity. See yourself as you want to be one year from now, with all the knowledge, experiences, and wisdom gained through this creation process. Imagine: You are that person now. You have been feeling and functioning this way for months now.

I'm so grateful that ...

I'm so freaking grateful for ...

Gratitude creates magic. Believe in it.

Example: *I'm so grateful that I am a person who loves to get up every morning and goes outside with a glass of water and sets intentions for my day. I am so freaking grateful I love to ride my bike and go for hikes. I am so grateful I am able to learn every day, because I am passionate about learning and seeking new knowledge and experiences. It makes me feel alive, and it allows me to help others. I value my friendships and connections with people who are authentic ...*

Create a Strategy for Your Vision to Become a Reality

You've crafted a clear vision of the vibrant health you desire. Now, it's time to bridge that vision with purposeful action by breaking it down into specific, achievable steps.

You can have the best vision and intentions, but they're empty without crafting a specific plan of *how* to manifest them in the real world. Having an intention to improve your cardiovascular health and sitting at home all day munching on chips will not get you to your goal, no matter how strong your intention is. There is an obvious conflict.

Use the guide below to create the necessary action steps to get where you want to go. Take each goal and think of the behaviors you must do consistently in order to achieve the goal.

Tip for Setting Goals

If you have long-term goals, that's great—keep them! I just have one suggestion: It may be helpful to break them down into smaller, short-term goals. Experiment with setting a smaller timeline; it may be easier to achieve a goal in a week or a month rather than a year. Break down the goal into daily and weekly goals.

1. Be simple and specific.

Make this new behavior so simple that you do not have to think about it too much. Be very specific about the action. If you come up with many action steps to reach your goal, that's great, but choose to do one to three steps at a time daily. Add a new step when the first one becomes a habit.

Example: I want to improve my bone and muscle strength to be able to live a healthy independent life (my why). I will put on my weighted backpack and go for a twenty-minute brisk walk every day.

2. Anchor it.

Anchor this new behavior to a habit you already have. Connecting something new with something you're already doing at a specific time will make it easier to follow through.

Example: *I'll take my backpack walk with my dogs right after lunch.* (This is my simple, specific, anchored-to-lunch action step I do daily.)

3. Repeat.

There is no magic formula for creating a habit. Repetition is what creates a habit. That's all. Changing habits is hard, but you can do it with a smart plan. You are where you are because of what you've repeated for years. Now it's time to repeat the new action step until it becomes a new, healthier habit.

Specific, Simple, and Anchored Habits to Inspire You

Not sure where to start? Here are some ideas of habits and anchor points to get you thinking:

- I only check social media when I am on the treadmill in the morning.
- After I go to the bathroom, I do push-ups and squats— as many as I can.
- After I get out of bed, I drink thirty-two ounces of water while I stand outside in the sunlight and set an intention for my day.
- I do ten squats and ten push-ups while waiting for the water to boil for my morning tea.
- After I eat dinner, I turn off all the overhead lights.
- After I sit down to eat, I take three deep breaths and express gratitude for my food.

- After I finish lunch, I take my dogs for a walk.
- After I eat dinner, I brush my teeth.
- I read news after my morning exercise.
- I drink my coffee after breakfast.
- After I finish work, I take a ten-minute walk around my neighborhood before starting dinner preparations.
- Every time I finish a phone call, I do a quick five-minute stretching routine.
- When I feel the urge to snack, I first drink a glass of water with lemon, mint, or apple cider vinegar.
- After brushing my teeth at night, I spend five minutes doing deep breathing exercises to relax and prepare for sleep.
- Every hour at work, I stand up and do a set of desk exercises, like leg lifts or arm circles, to keep active throughout the day.
- I end my shower in the morning with cold water.
- I eat a bowl of vegetables with each main meal.

Oh, and every day I do at least one thing that brings me joy. And so should you!

Change Your Environment

Changing your environment can significantly impact your ability to achieve health goals. Sometimes we must alter our environment in order to develop healthy habits. Below are some examples of specific statements and commitments you can make to change your environment for the better:

- I don't keep cookies in the house, only low-glycemic fruits.

- I remove chairs from my office so there's only one option—to stand.
- I hire a trainer to do resistance training three times a week.
- I place water pitchers in multiple locations around my home to remind me to stay hydrated.
- I keep dumbbells, resistance bands, or yoga mats in my living room for easy access to quick workouts.
- I keep my vegetables at eye level, washed and cut in the refrigerator, ready to eat.
- I only keep real, whole foods in the house.
- I keep healthy cookbooks on my kitchen counter for inspiration and easy access.
- I install blue-light filters on my devices to reduce eye strain and improve sleep quality.
- I subscribe to a healthy meal delivery service (such as Daily Harvest, Trifecta, Blue Apron, Green Chef, or Daily Dose).
- I create a sleep-friendly environment by using blackout curtains and a comfortable organic mattress.
- I add plants to my home to create a calming atmo-sphere with cleaner air.

Commit to Yourself

Now that you have a clear vision, dedicate time each morning and night to focusing on your vision. Feel it, and believe it as you read the statements you've constructed aloud or silently. This is the practice of focusing on what you want. This part is very important so that you are not subconsciously running through your old thoughts; rather, you are changing your thoughts and emotions with daily reading and visualizing. Consistency and belief are key to success.

Ride Some Brain Waves

I've mentioned in previous chapters that I enjoy listening to theta-wave frequencies while meditating. I also listen to them through my headphones while reading and imagining my vision every day; this practice can be profoundly impactful. You may remember from our chapter on sleep that theta waves occur just as you're drifting off to sleep, entering that deeply imaginative state right before the deep, delta-wave sleep takes over. This stage is ripe for suggestions, making your mind exceptionally open to new ideas. This is the imaginative, hypnotic mind.

Again, I recommend downloading an app with binaural beats, and set it to theta waves, put on headphones, and see your life the way you desire. You have power over your destiny.

Identify the Support You Need

We have greater chances of success when we have support from people in our lives. When you want to transform your health, you're the only one responsible for your results. No one can force you to go to the gym, no one can demand that you eat more vegetables, no one can make you stop using plastic water bottles. No one will know if you actually did fifty push-ups, and no one will be aware if you actually did your visualization exercise last night.

This is why it's a good idea to have someone hold you accountable to your goals. Share your new goals with your family. Tell your best friend to call you to make sure you went for that morning walk. Hire a coach for support. Be honest about what help and support you need to succeed—and ask for it.

Be Conscious of Your Relationships

There will inevitably be times when there's conflict between your goals and your social life. Here are some tips for making the right decisions:

- **Share your health goals openly and honestly.** Clarify your reasons for making healthier choices with your loved ones. When talking to family and friends about goals, explain how their support, or lack of it, affects you. Use "I feel" statements to express how you feel when your choices are unsupported or criticized. Be specific about what types of support you need.

- **Reevaluate relationships and find a supportive community.** If certain people don't support you, or even show interest in your goals, it may be necessary to question their role in your life. Seek out like-minded individuals or communities who share your health goals and can offer the encouragement you need. Find a workout buddy or participate in group coaching sessions where you can connect with others with shared goals.

- **Focus on your goals.** Make yourself the priority rather than trying to change your spouse or friends. This is self-love, giving yourself the gift of health.

Approach with Confidence and Patience

Contrary to popular belief, people aren't born confident. They learn to believe in themselves through trial and error, through falls and victories. In short, confidence simply comes from the process of doing—whatever that may be.

Setbacks are inevitable; no human can avoid them. But the lessons we learn from these challenges are invaluable. Both you and I have gained confidence in many aspects of life because we chose to confront and overcome difficulties. Transformation, of course, demands a balance of confidence and humility. Humility teaches us to ask for help, learn from experiences, and adapt our strategies as needed. It empowers us to rise after a fall, recognizing our limitations without self-judgment. This ability to embrace imperfection and continue moving forward is, in itself, a profound transformation.

It's natural to want results immediately, or "soon," but it doesn't work like that in most cases. The most important things in life require time and hard work, which inherently involves patience. Have patience. Getting started toward your vision is the toughest part, but once you take the first step, you'll build momentum. And from there you won't stop until you finish. Trust me—I believe in you!

Avoid Making Excuses

My clients have different goals: to feel better in their bodies, to gain more energy, to sleep better, to eat healthier, to lose weight, and so on. What most of them have in common is waiting for the perfect time to start their journey.

You've heard it before:

"I'll take care of myself when I have more money."

"I'll begin when my son goes to college."

"I'll start when my husband is out of town."

"I'll find time when I'm done with that project at work."

This is just procrastination, plain and simple.

If you're waiting for that magical moment to start your health transformation, let's be honest—you're not in the right mindset. It's time to dig deep and confront the fears holding you back from a healthier life. Ask yourself why it's easier for you to prioritize work, family, and other things more than yourself. Your life is happening right now as you are reading these words. Don't wait until it is too late.

It may be time to take a moment to look inside yourself. If you truly want to improve your health, there is no better day than today. There will never be a perfect time when the skies open up and light beams down, compelling you to buy organic food or go for a walk.

Start now. Take a small yet significant step. You won't always be able to give 100 percent, and that's okay—as long as you show up. All it takes is one tiny step, like drinking more water or doing one push-up. Start today.

Trust the Process

Through all my falls and adversity, I've learned one beautiful lesson that makes my life so much easier now: When things don't work out as I planned, I trust there is something better. Sometimes my mind may be limited in seeing what's possible, what can truly be the best outcome.

When you believe in the highest good being created for you, in the universe, that your inner light knows what's meant for you and what's best for you, that's what guides you on your journey.

Instead of getting frustrated or pushing and forcing things I want, I know when to let go and feel grateful for the powerful, unseen guidance I receive.

Trust the process. Every day take one simple step at a time, and your health goals will fall into place.

Plan for Obstacles

Your path to healthy change will inevitably include roadblocks and potential pitfalls. Take it easy on yourself. Everyone stumbles. Just keep showing up! Acknowledge the big rock in the road. Celebrate something about yourself and start again.

When you're doing something new, it will involve some degree of difficulty. If you emphasize how tough it is, you'll make it that much more challenging. Instead, focus on elements of the experience you enjoy: breathing in the fresh air, chopping vegetables, choosing new workout gear. Overall, always focus on your desire and your *why*.

Sometimes it's helpful to also ask yourself questions like these:

- Where do I fear ending up if I do nothing?
- What could I imagine doing if I knew I could only succeed with this new habit?

Let the answers guide you.

I'll share my experience of going through this process as an example. I do not enjoy high-intensity training, though I know it is essential to do it once a week for my cardiovascular health. I want a healthy heart. So I think about how I feel after the exercise. That gets me to perform it with more excitement. I don't think about the training; I think about the incredible feeling of joy and the proud moment of accomplishment. The other important part is, it's on my calendar for every Saturday. Nonnegotiable. Every Saturday morning, I get on my Peloton bike and do a high-intensity Norwegian 4x4 bike ride. And I really do feel amazing after I do it.

Ideas if You're Struggling to Return to Healthy Habits

Because this will be a repetitive process, here are my best ideas to return to as you set yourself up for success:

Plan

If you know something will soon disrupt your routine, have a plan for that time period. Include all the things you prioritize so you don't have to fall off your routine. Have some flexibility for unexpected situations.

Communicate

If possible, communicate with everyone involved. For example, when my life coach visited us from New York, she communicated clearly that her routine was to walk on the treadmill in the morning. I knew not to interrupt her. Whatever it is, whether it's your meditation or your run between 6 and 7 a.m., let everyone know. It's important to care for yourself first.

Be Flexible

Whatever happens, don't completely stop your new healthy habits. Try to adjust the timing or the activity. If you do need to make a change, I recommend modifying the routine to make it fit into your holiday or other life event. I do not recommend cutting it out 100 percent, as doing so will become a pattern of stopping and starting, making it more challenging to start again every time.

If you have truly developed a habit, like drinking water in the morning, viewing sunlight, eating your last meal at 5 p.m., or doing yoga every day, you'll keep at it most of the time, if not all of the time. Speaking from my own experience, there isn't a morning where I don't drink my thirty-two ounces of water, stand in the morning light setting an intention for my day, do some body movement like Qigong or yoga, and read my vision. These activities are who I am. Just as you drink your coffee and read the news no matter where you are, you can incorporate daily habits that transform your health.

Summary: From Vision to Reality

1. **Set a clear vision** for your health and life.
2. **Know the why** of your vision.
3. **Break it into specific, achievable steps.** Take small actions daily.
4. **Anchor new habits** to existing ones.
5. **Repeat the new behavior daily.**
6. **Seek support** and accountability.
7. **Plan for obstacles** and stay focused on your **why**.
8. **Trust the process.** Consistency, belief, and patience are key.

Transformation is within your reach. Take one small step today and trust that every action brings you closer to the vibrant health and life you desire.

As we come to the end of this journey together, I want to take a moment to reflect on everything we've covered. We've delved into a wealth of information about your external and inner environment, food as nutrition, the importance of sleep and everyday movement, and how all this connects to the health of the dream team M&M, which is the foundation of you feeling, functioning, and looking great.

Hopefully, all this ignited a spark of inspiration within you. This book has been a roadmap, but now it's up to you to take the wheel and drive toward a healthier, more vibrant life.

Remember, there is nothing more important than your health. Our health starts in our mind—how we think about health and our lifestyle. When you truly take ownership of your health and decide that nothing can get in the way, that's when real change happens. Make this decision every morning when you rise and each night before you sleep. This journey to living well doesn't end here—it starts now.

Don't just move on after reading this book—take action! Implement the habits, tips, and strategies we've discussed. Make a plan to incorporate these changes into your daily life. Start with small, manageable steps and build from there. Every choice you make, no matter how small, moves you closer to the vibrant health and well-being you deserve.

Like mastering an instrument, cooking, or playing a sport, excelling in anything new requires willingness and commitment to show up and practice consistently. This principle applies equally to health and realizing any vision.

My hope is that this book will help you take charge of your health. I want you to let go of the stories of the past and focus on your created vision of feeling, functioning, and looking the way you have dreamed. You deserve it, and you can have it!

If you ever feel lost or need guidance along the way, don't hesitate to reach out to me via my website.[121] Seeking support is a sign of strength. Hire the right functional medicine team to guide and support you. Surround yourself with people who uplift you, empower you, and support you.

You have the power to transform your life. Embrace this journey with determination and enthusiasm. Set your goals, make a plan, and take the first step today. Your future self will thank you for the commitment and effort you put in now.

It's your turn to build the life you envision. Let your journey be a testament to the incredible strength and resilience within you. Here's to your health, happiness, and a life filled with endless possibilities. Go out there and live well!

READER'S GUIDE

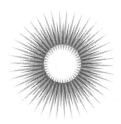

CHAPTER ONE
UNDERSTANDING AND ELIMINATING ENVIRONMENTAL TOXINS

This book is about more than just physical well-being; it's about cultivating resilience, vitality, and a balanced lifestyle that encompasses the mind, body, and spirit. Understanding your body's needs and your environment is crucial in shaping a fulfilling life where you wake up each day feeling energized, with the mental clarity to handle life's challenges.

Discussion Questions

1. What are mitochondria, and how do they impact your daily energy levels?
2. Reflect on how mitochondria function as cellular powerhouses and what they need to keep you

energized. How does your microbiome contribute to your overall health?

3. Consider the role of the microbiome in digestion, immunity, and even mood regulation. What are the consequences of neglecting your mitochondria and microbiome?

4. Identify symptoms like fatigue, brain fog, or weight gain that may signal dysfunction in these systems.

5. Reflect on the synergy between mitochondria and the microbiome in promoting overall health. How do mitochondria and the microbiome work together for optimal wellness?

6. Think about your diet, sleep habits, stress levels, and how they support or hinder these two systems. What daily lifestyle choices affect your mitochondria and microbiome?

7. What are some toxins that disrupt the function of mitochondria and the microbiome, and how can you avoid them? Explore ways to minimize exposure to environmental toxins and processed foods.

Journal

What specific change will you implement this week to better support your mitochondria and microbiome?

Understanding and caring for your mitochondria and microbiome is key to creating lasting health and vitality. These two systems, though microscopic, have a profound impact on every aspect of your well-being—from energy production to health to immune support and beyond. By making intentional choices to nourish and protect them, you empower yourself to live with greater energy, clarity, and resilience. Small steps toward healthier food choices, toxin elimination, and stress reduction can lead to significant improvements in how you feel and function each day.

CHAPTER TWO
THE POWER OF REAL, WHOLE FOODS

This chapter explores the comprehensive role that food plays in our health and well-being, emphasizing not just **what** we eat, but also **when, how,** and **how much** we eat. This chapter underscores the importance of distinguishing between real, whole foods and ultraprocessed factory foods, highlighting how these choices impact our energy levels, overall health, and risk of chronic disease. Through stories, this chapter illustrates the transformative power of nutrition when combined with mindful eating practices.

Discussion Questions
Understanding Food Choices

1. What are the key differences between real, whole foods and ultraprocessed factory foods as outlined in this chapter? How do these differences impact our health on a daily basis?

2. Reflect on your own daily food choices. How much of your diet is made up of real, whole foods versus ultraprocessed foods? What changes could you make to improve your dietary habits?

The Importance of Protein

3. This chapter discusses the importance of protein in our diets. What role does protein play in maintaining

health, and why is it essential to get the right balance of amino acids?

4. How do you currently ensure you're getting enough protein in your diet? Are there any adjustments you need to make to meet your body's needs?

Meal Timing and Biological Clock

5. This chapter emphasizes the importance of aligning meal times with our natural biological clock. How does meal timing affect digestion and overall health?

6. Reflect on your eating habits. Do you typically eat late at night or skip meals? How might changing your meal timing improve your health?

Personalization and Testing

7. This chapter highlights the importance of personalized nutrition and testing (e.g., genetic testing, continuous glucose monitoring). Why is it important to tailor your diet to your unique biology?

8. Have you ever considered or tried personalized nutrition strategies? What were your experiences, and how did they influence your understanding of your body's needs?

Summer's Story

9. Summer's story is a powerful example of personalized health care. How did understanding her genetic makeup and specific needs lead to a significant improvement in her health?

10. In what ways can Summer's story inspire others to take control of their health, especially when dealing with chronic or mysterious health issues?

Taking Action

11. After reading this chapter, what is one specific change you plan to make in your food choices or lifestyle to improve your health? What steps will you take to implement this change?

12. How can you apply the principles from this chapter to support the health and well-being of your family or community?

Journal

Consider keeping a food journal for a week, as suggested in the chapter. Afterward, ask yourself: What insights did I gain from this practice? How did it affect my understanding of my eating habits and their impact on my health?

CHAPTER THREE
TRANSFORMING YOUR ENERGY THROUGH SLEEP

This chapter delves into the critical role of sleep in our health and well-being. It emphasizes that sleep is not just a passive time of rest, but an active process where the body heals, detoxifies, and rejuvenates itself. This chapter highlights the importance of both the quantity and quality of sleep, explaining how poor sleep habits can lead to a cascade of health issues, from weakened immunity to difficulty in managing daily tasks, regulating emotions, and maintaining physical health.

Discussion Questions

Understanding Sleep's Role

1. What are the key functions of sleep as described in this chapter? How does sleep contribute to both physical and mental health?

2. Reflect on your own sleep habits. How do you feel when you don't get enough sleep? How does it impact your daily life and health?

The Importance of a Sleep Routine

3. This chapter emphasizes the importance of a consistent sleep routine. Why is going to bed and waking up at the same time each day so crucial for sleep quality? How does understanding the circadian rhythm change your perspective on sleep?

4. What challenges do you face in maintaining a consistent sleep schedule? What strategies could help you overcome these challenges?

Sleep and Overall Health

5. How does poor sleep contribute to other health issues, such as weight gain, weakened immunity, or mental health challenges?

6. How might improving your sleep positively impact other areas of your health and life?

Creating a Sleep-Friendly Environment

7. This chapter discusses the importance of a sleep-friendly environment. What are some ways you can create a better sleep environment in your bedroom?

8. How can you minimize disruptions to your sleep, such as noise, light, or electronic devices?

Behavior Change and Commitment

9. This chapter suggests that committing to a consistent sleep routine helps to create long-term health. What specific changes are you willing to make to improve your sleep? What are your long-term health goals, and how can improving your sleep contribute to achieving them?

10. How can you hold yourself accountable for maintaining these changes over time?

Personal Reflection

11. Think about a time when you were sleep-deprived. How did it affect your mood, productivity, and overall health? What did you learn from that experience?

12. How does this chapter inspire you to view sleep as a nonnegotiable part of your health routine?

Taking Action

13. After reading this chapter, what is one specific action you plan to take to improve your sleep? How will you incorporate this into your daily routine?

14. How can you support your family or household in adopting healthier sleep habits?

Journal

Consider keeping a sleep journal for a week, as suggested in the chapter. Afterward, reflect: What insights did you gain from tracking your sleep? How did it affect your understanding of the relationship between your sleep patterns and overall well-being?

CHAPTER FOUR
BUILDING STRONG HEALTH
THROUGH MOVEMENT

This chapter emphasizes the vital role of movement in maintaining a healthy body and mind. It challenges the notion that exercise is simply a means to lose weight or build muscle, instead presenting movement as an essential daily activity that supports overall health, prevents chronic diseases, and enhances mental well-being. Through relatable stories and practical tips, the chapter encourages readers to view movement as a joyful and necessary part of life. It also provides guidance on how to integrate regular, intentional movement into even the busiest schedules.

Discussion Questions
Understanding the Importance of Movement

1. What are the key benefits of regular movement as described in the chapter? How does movement impact both physical and mental health?

2. Reflect on your current level of daily movement. How do you feel when you are active versus when you are sedentary?

Making Movement a Habit

3. This chapter suggests incorporating at least thirty minutes of intentional movement into your daily routine. What challenges might you face in achieving this goal?

4. What strategies can you use to ensure you make time for movement every day, even on busy days?

Movement and Mental Health

5. How does regular movement contribute to better mental health, according to this chapter? Have you noticed any changes in your mood or stress levels after being physically active?

6. How can you use movement as a tool to manage stress and improve your overall mental well-being?

Personalizing Your Movement Routine

7. This chapter emphasizes finding movement activities that you enjoy. What types of movement do you find most enjoyable, and how can you incorporate them into your life regularly?

8. How does personalizing your movement routine make it more sustainable and enjoyable over the long term?

Behavior Change and Accountability

9. How do tools like these help in forming new habits and staying consistent?

10. Have you used similar tools before? If so, how effective were they in helping you maintain a regular movement routine?

Taking Action

11. After reading this chapter, what is one specific action you plan to take to increase your daily movement? How will you incorporate this into your routine?

12. How can you encourage your family or friends to join you in becoming more active?

Journal

Consider keeping a movement journal for a week, as suggested in the chapter. Afterward, reflect: What insights did you gain from tracking your physical activity? How did it affect your understanding of the relationship between movement and your overall well-being?

CHAPTER 5
INNER ENVIRONMENT

This chapter explores the profound connection between emotional health and physical health, with a personal narrative illustrating how unresolved trauma can manifest as physical symptoms. It underscores the importance of addressing emotional pain, practicing mindfulness, and nurturing your inner environment through various practices like meditation, journaling, and connecting with nature.

Discussion Questions
The Connection Between Inner and Outer Health

1. How has your inner environment (thoughts, emotions, beliefs) affected your physical health? Can you identify any connections between unresolved emotional issues and physical symptoms you've experienced?

2. How do you currently manage the negative emotions that arise from your inner environment? Reflect on the strategies you use to cope with stress, anxiety, or unresolved trauma. Are these strategies effective, or

do they merely suppress your emotions? How can you begin to address these emotions in a healthier way?

Influence of Environment on Well-Being

3. In what ways do your external environment and relationships influence your inner environment? Consider the people, places, and situations that surround you daily. How do they impact your thoughts, emotions, and overall well-being? What changes can you make in your external environment to better support your inner health?

Awareness and Transformation for Inner Growth

4. The chapter emphasizes the importance of becoming aware of your inner environment. What practices, such as journaling or meditation, can you incorporate into your daily routine to support this awareness?
5. Reflect on the idea of transforming your identity to support better health. What negative beliefs or narratives about yourself would you like to change, and how can you start shifting them today?

Learning from the Author's Healing Journey

6. The author shares her journey of healing from emotional trauma. How does her experience resonate with you, and what lessons can you take away to apply to your own healing journey?

Journal

Take a moment to reflect on the connection between your inner and outer environments. How have past experiences shaped your current state of mind and health? As you move forward, focus on becoming more aware of the thoughts, emotions, and beliefs that shape your inner environment. Make a commitment to daily practices that nurture your mental and emotional well-being, such as meditation, journaling, or connecting with nature. Remember, transformation begins from within, and by cultivating a healthier inner environment, you can profoundly impact your physical health and overall quality of life.

CHAPTER SIX
TRANSFORMATION

The final chapter outlines a practical and philosophical approach to transformation, detailing six core principles: openness, honesty, willingness, patience, commitment, and consistency. It encourages readers to cultivate awareness, follow their intuition, redefine their identity, create a vision, and commit to their goals with a step-by-step strategy. It provides a comprehensive guide to achieving personal transformation by redefining your identity and embracing new, healthier habits.

Discussion Questions
Mindset and Motivation

1. How does this chapter suggest you shift your mindset to support transformation? What are some examples from your own life where a mindset shift led to significant change?

Understanding Identity

2. The chapter discusses the concept of identity as how you perceive yourself in the present moment. What

are some limiting beliefs or self-descriptions you currently hold? How might these be redefined to support your transformation goals?

The Role of Patience

3. This chapter emphasizes the need for patience in the transformation process. How do you balance the desire for immediate results with the understanding that true transformation takes time?

Practical Exercises

4. This chapter includes practical exercises for creating a new identity and vision. Which exercise resonated with you the most, and how do you plan to implement it in your daily routine?

Handling Setbacks

5. Transformation often involves setbacks. What strategies does the chapter offer for overcoming obstacles, and how can you apply these to challenges you currently face?

Support Systems

6. How important is having a support system in your transformation journey? What role do your current relationships play in your ability to achieve your goals, and how might you seek additional support if needed?

Trusting the Process

7. This chapter concludes with the idea of trusting yourself and the process of transformation. How do you
currently view your ability to trust in your journey, and
what practices could enhance this trust?

Journal

*Reflect on your current journey toward transformation. Consider
what aspects of your identity, habits, or mindset might be
holding you back and how you can apply the principles from
this chapter to create lasting, meaningful change in your life.*

ACKNOWLEDGMENTS

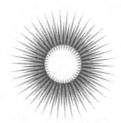

First and foremost, I am deeply grateful to my clients, friends, and family who entrusted me with their hopes and allowed me the privilege of guiding them. Your belief in me has been the foundation of this work.

I also want to express my sincere thanks to the doctors, scientists, and passionate individuals in holistic health. Your teachings through books, talks, and seminars have been invaluable in shaping my understanding and approach to functional medicine, biohacking, and achieving vibrant health.

I would like to specifically acknowledge the mentors, coaches, guides, and writers in my personal, business, and health development who have guided me, often without even knowing: Dr. Dan Kalish, Dr. Bruce Lipton, PhD, Dr. Rhonda Patrick, Dr. Joe Dispenza, Dr. Gabrielle Lyon, Dr. Ben Lynch, Dr. Joseph Mercola, Dr. Peter Attia, Dr. Mark Hyman, Dr. Mindy Pelz, Dr. Casey Means, Dr. Carrie Jones, Dr. Elaine Aron, Dr.

Paul Conti, Dr. Richard Schwartz, Dave Asprey, Donald Miller, Seth Godin, Tony Robbins, Ben Greenfield, Gabby Bernstein, Gary Zukav, Eri Kardos, and Lauren Zander—your work has profoundly impacted my life, and I hope this book will do the same for others.

To my fellow authors, I now fully appreciate the journey of bringing a book to life. It is both challenging and rewarding, not just to research, study, and write but to ensure this work reaches those who need it most. I am grateful for the incredible support team that made the sharing of this book possible on a much larger scale—Brand Builders Group, Mission Driven Press, and Forefront Books. Without you, this project would not have reached those it's meant to help.

A special thanks to all my dear friends for your love and unwavering support and belief in my work. Your insight and encouragement in my life have been invaluable.

A big thank-you to Miriam Carbo for the beautiful food photography and for making the entire process so enjoyable.

To my husband, Mark: Your support for everything I embark on—regardless of the outcome—has always meant the world to me. You see my passion, my dedication to others, and you are always there to cheer me on.

To my daughter, Summer Faith, my HSP, whose wisdom and spirit challenge and inspire me daily. You've shaped me into a better person, filling my heart with love and making me laugh and cry like no one else. Thank you for helping with the recipes, illustrations, and design, and being my sounding board.

To everyone who believed in me and supported this work, whether mentioned by name or not, thank you from the bottom of my heart.

If this book changes just one life in a big, beautiful way, it was worth every moment.

NOTES

1 Chris Dawson, "Genetics Affects Functions of the Gut Microbiome," Cornell Chronicle, April 18, 2022, https://news.cornell.edu/stories/2022/04/genetics-affects-functions-gut-microbiome.

2 FDA, GRAS Final Rule, 21 CFR 170.30

3 Vinay M. Pathak et al., " Current status of pesticide effects on environment, human health and its eco-friendly management as bioremediation: A comprehensive review," Journal Frontiers in Microbiology, no. 13 (2022), https://pmc.ncbi.nlm.nih.gov/articles/PMC9428564/.

4 "Survey: 40% of Americans' Daily Lives Are Disrupted by Digestive Troubles," EndoProMag, April 15, 2023, https://www.endopromag.com/survey-40-of-americans-daily-lives-are-disrupted-by-digestive-troubles/.

5 "The Top 10 Most Common Chronic Conditions in Older Adults," National Council on Aging, October 22, 2021, https://www.ncoa.org/article/the-top-10-most-common-chronic-conditions-in-older-adults/.

6 "Alcohol Is One of the Biggest Risk Factors for Breast Cancer," WHO News, October 20, 2021, https://www.who.int/europe/news/item/20-10-2021-alcohol-is-one-of-the-biggest-risk-factors-for-breast-cancer.

7 "Added Sugar Repository," Hypoglycemia.org, https://hypoglycemia.org/added-sugar-repository/.

8 Iqbal Pittalwala,"Widely Consumed Vegetable Oil Leads to Unhealthy Gut," UC Riverside News, July 3, 2023, https://news.ucr.edu/articles/2023/07/03/widely-consumed-vegetable-oil-leads-unhealthy-gut.

9 Jules Bernstein, "America's Most Widely Consumed Oil Causes Genetic Changes in Brain," UC Riverside News, January 17, 2020, https://news.ucr.edu/articles/2020/01/17/americas-most-widely-consumed-oil-causes-genetic-changes-brain.

10 Trasias Mukama et al., "IGF-1 and Risk of Morbidity and Mortality from

Cancer, Cardiovascular Diseases, and All Causes in EPIC-Heidelberg," The Journal of Clinical Endocrinology & Metabolism 108, no. 10 (2023): e1092–e1102, https://academic.oup.com/jcem/article/108/10/e1092/7124430?login=false.

11 Asghar Ali et al., "Pesticides: Unintended Impact on the Hidden World of Gut Microbiota," Metabolites 14, no. 3 (2024), https://pmc.ncbi.nlm.nih.gov/articles/PMC10971818/.

12 Tasha Stoiber, PhD, "What Are Parabens?" Environmental Working Group, April 9, 2019, https://www.ewg.org/what-are-parabens.

13 Jonathan Vellinga, "Leaky Gut Syndrome May Be the Cause of Your Brain Health Issues," Temecula Center for Integrative Medicine, December 10, 2020, https://www.tcimedicine.com/post/leaky-gut-syndrome-may-be-the-cause-of-your-brain-health-issues.

14 Alessio Fasano, "All disease begins in the (leaky) gut: role of zonulin-mediated gut permeability in the pathogenesis of some chronic inflammatory diseases," F1000Res 9, (2020), https://pmc.ncbi.nlm.nih.gov/articles/PMC6996528/.

15 "Acrylamide and Cancer Risk," American Cancer Society, 2023, https://www.cancer.org/cancer/risk-prevention/chemicals/acrylamide.html.

16 Rekhadevi Perumalla Venkata et al., " Evaluation of the deleterious health effects of consumption of repeatedly heated vegetable oil," Toxicology reports 3, (2016), https://pmc.ncbi.nlm.nih.gov/articles/PMC5616019/.

17 Xuhui Chen et al., "Adverse effects of triclosan exposure on health and potential molecular mechanisms," The Science of the total environment 879, (2023), https://pmc.ncbi.nlm.nih.gov/articles/PMC10035793/.

18 Filippo Acconcia et al., "Molecular Mechanisms of Action of BPA," Dose-response: a publication of International Hormesis Society, no. 4 (2015), https://pmc.ncbi.nlm.nih.gov/articles/PMC4679188/.

19 Raffaele Marfella, MD, PhD, et al., "Microplastics and Nanoplastics in Atheromas and Cardiovascular Events," The New England Journal of Medicine 390, no. 10 (2024), https://www.nejm.org/doi/full/10.1056/NEJMoa2309822.

20 Ketura Persellin, "Pervasive Phthalates: New Study Links Child Exposure to Cancer," EWG News & Insights, March 24, 2022, https://www.ewg.org/

news-insights/news/2022/03/pervasive-phthalates-new-study-links-child-exposure-cancer.

21 Vera Dias, et al., "The Role of Oxidative Stress in Parkinson's Disease," National Library of Medicine, August 18, 2014, https://pmc.ncbi.nlm.nih.gov/articles/PMC4135313/.

22 L. B. Miller et al., "Impact of exposure to per- and polyfluoroalkyl substances on fecal microbiota composition in mother-infant dyads," medRxiv, December 14, 2022, https://www.medrxiv.org/content/10.1101/2022.12.14.22283359v1.full.

23 Get your guide to healthy eating out at https://yourwellness-madesimple.com/shop/.

24 Beverly Merz, "Sauna Use Linked to Longer Life, Fewer Fatal Heart Problems," Harvard Health Blog, February 25, 2015, https://www.health.harvard.edu/blog/sauna-use-linked-longer-life-fewer-fatal-heart-problems-201502257755.

25 Kelly K. McCann, MD, "Health Benefits of Sauna Use," Dr. Kelly McCann, https://drkellymccann.com/health-benefits-of-sauna-use/.

26 "Prediabetes: Could It Be You?" CDC, 2023, https://www.cdc.gov/diabetes/communication-resources/prediabetes-statistics.html.

27 "What you should know about processed, ultra-processed foods," Mayo Clinic Health System, July 25, 2024, https://www.mayoclinichealthsystem.org/hometown-health/speaking-of-health/processed-foods-what-you-should-know.

28 Monica Dus, "What You Eat Can Reprogram Your Genes," ASBMB Today, March 27, 2022. https://www.asbmb.org/asbmb-today/science/032722/what-you-eat-can-reprogram-your-genes.

29 Elena A. Ponomarenko et al., "The Size of the Human Proteome: The Width and Depth," National Library of Medicine, May 19, 2016, https://pmc.ncbi.nlm.nih.gov/articles/PMC4889822/.

30 Stephanie Eckelkamp, "How much protein do I need, and how do I get enough?" Levels, July 25, 2023, https://www.levels.com/blog/how-much-protein-do-i-need-and-how-do-i-get-enough.

31 Rosanna Chianese et al.,"Impact of Dietary Fats on Brain Functions," Curr Neuropharmacol, no. 7 (2018), https://pmc.ncbi.nlm.nih.gov/articles/PMC6120115/.

32 T. S. Sathyanarayana et al., "Understanding Nutrition, Depression and Mental Illnesses," Indian Journal of Psychiatry 50, no. 2 (2008), https://pmc.ncbi.nlm.nih.gov/articles/PMC2738337/?_kx=dRoo4q9riTqul3z-rAZDDXTmIJrlD5Bo-FslGgCw7zjA%3D.HKMsXE.

33 Kathryn A. Wierenga et al., "Omega-3 Fatty Acids And Inflammation—You Are What You Eat!" Frontiers for young minds 9, (2020), https://pmc.ncbi.nlm.nih.gov/articles/PMC8846546/.

34 Dr. Jennie Stanford, "Insulin Resistance and Inflammation: Understanding the Connection," Rupa Health, September 17, 2024, https://www.rupahealth.com/post/insulin-resistance-and-inflammation-understanding-the-connection.

35 Brett Smiley, "How Much Fiber Should I Eat Per Day?" Healthline, May 30, 2023, https://www.healthline.com/health/food-nutrition/how-much-fiber-per-day.

36 Anthropological studies show that historically, humans consumed more fiber than what we do now in the modern world. Our hunter-gatherer ancestors typically ate around 100 grams of fiber a day from eating a lot of plant such as vegetables, fruits, tubers, nuts and seeds.

37 Jingjing Kang et al., "Butyrate ameliorates colorectal cancer through regulating intestinal microecological disorders," Anti-cancer drugs 34, no. 2 (2023): 227-237, https://pmc.ncbi.nlm.nih.gov/articles/PMC9815807/.

38 Sandy Cohen, "If you want to boost immunity, look to the gut," UCLA Health, March 19, 2021, https://www.uclahealth.org/news/article/want-to-boost-immunity-look-to-the-gut.

39 "Study shows how serotonin and a popular anti-depressant affect the gut's microbiota," ScienceDaily, September 6, 2019, https://www.sciencedaily.com/releases/2019/09/190906092809.htm.

40 "More than 90 percent of soybean, cotton, and corn acres planted by U.S. farmers use genetically engineered seeds," USDA Economic Research Service, October 7, 2024, https://www.ers.usda.gov/data-products/charts-of-note/charts-of-note/?topicId=a2d1ab41-13b3-48b5-8451-688d73507ff4.

41 Janelle Weaver, "Fermented-food diet increases microbiome diversity, decreases inflammatory proteins, study finds," Stanford Medicine, July

12, 2021, https://med.stanford.edu/news/all-news/2021/07/fermented-food-diet-increases-microbiome-diversity-lowers-inflammation.

42 Ben Lynch, "Histamine Intolerance: How It May Be Affecting You," SeekingHealth, June 30, 2021, https://www.seekinghealth.com/blogs/education/dgp-episode-14-histamine-intolerance.

43 Kaijian Hou et al., "Microbiota in health and diseases," Sig Transduct Target Ther 7, no. 135 (2022), https://www.nature.com/articles/s41392-022-00974-4.

44 Jan Triska et al., "Factors Influencing Sulforaphane Content in Broccoli Sprouts and Subsequent Sulforaphane Extraction," Foods (Basel, Switzerland) 10, no. 8 (2021), https://pmc.ncbi.nlm.nih.gov/articles/PMC8394606/.

45 Liping Guo et al., "Effect of freezing methods on sulforaphane formation in broccoli sprouts," RSC Advances 5 (2015), https://pubs.rsc.org/en/content/articlehtml/2015/ra/c5ra03403e.

46 Li Tang et al., "Intake of Cruciferous Vegetables Modifies Bladder Cancer Survival," Cancer Epidemiology, Biomarkers & Prevention 19, no. 7 (2010), https://www.ncbi.nlm.nih.gov/pmc/articles/PMC2901397/.

47 "Researchers Call Herbs Rich Source of Healthy Antioxidants; Oregano Ranks Highest," ScienceDaily, January 8, 2002, https://www.science-daily.com/releases/2002/01/020108075158.htm.

48 Ana Carolina Remondi Souza et al., "The Integral Role of Magnesium in Muscle Integrity and Aging: A Comprehensive Review," Nutrients 15, no. 24 (2023), https://pmc.ncbi.nlm.nih.gov/articles/PMC10745813/.

49 Roya Shabkhizan et al., "The Beneficial and Adverse Effects of Autophagic Response to Caloric Restriction and Fasting," Advances in nutrition (Bethesda, Md.) 14, no. 5 (2023): 1211–1225, https://pmc.ncbi.nlm.nih.gov/articles/PMC10509423/.

50 Hannaneh Parveresh et al., "Mechanistic Insights into Fasting-induced Autophagy in the Aging Heart," World Journal of Cardiology 16, no. 3 (2024): 109-117, https://pmc.ncbi.nlm.nih.gov/articles/PMC10989221/.

51 Emily Hobbs, "Fasting and Cancer: Can Fasting Really Help Fight the Disease?" Ezra, January 31, 2024, https://ezra.com/blog/fasting-and-cancer.

52 Basem H Elesawy et al., "The Impact of Intermittent Fasting on Brain-

Derived Neurotrophic Factor, Neurotrophin 3, and Rat Behavior in a Rat Model of Type 2 Diabetes Mellitus," Brain Sciences 11, no. 2 (2021), https://pmc.ncbi.nlm.nih.gov/articles/PMC7918995/.

53 Sneha Mishra et al., "Time-Restricted Eating and Its Metabolic Benefits," Journal of Clinical Medicine 12, no. 22 (2023): 7007, https://pmc.ncbi.nlm.nih.gov/articles/PMC10672223/.

54 Sara Lindberg, "Autophagy: What You Need to Know," Healthline, May 5, 2023, https://www.healthline.com/health/autophagy.

55 Caitlin Colling et al., "Changes in Serum Cortisol Levels After 10 Days of Overfeeding and Fasting," Endocrinology and Metabolism, May 23, 2023, https://journals.physiology.org/doi/full/10.1152/ajpendo.00181.2022.

56 Mariyam Khalid et al., "Advanced Glycation End Product and Diabetes Mellitus: Mechanisms and Perspectives," Biomolecules 12, no. 4 (2022), https://www.ncbi.nlm.nih.gov/pmc/articles/PMC9030615/.

57 Walter Gulisano et al., "Role of Amyloid-β and Tau Proteins in Alzheimer's Disease: Confuting the Amyloid Cascade," Journal of Alzheimer's Disease 64, suppl. 1 (2018), https://www.ncbi.nlm.nih.gov/pmc/articles/PMC8371153/.

58 Arthur José Pontes Oliveira de Almeida et al., "Unveiling the Role of Inflammation and Oxidative Stress on Age-Related Cardiovascular Diseases," Oxidative Medicine and Cellular Longevity 2020, (2020), https://www.ncbi.nlm.nih.gov/pmc/articles/PMC7232723/.

59 Katie Wells, "Does a Pressure Cooker Destroy Nutrients?" Wellness Mama, February 10, 2016, https://wellnessmama.com/natural-home/pressure-cooker-nutrients/.

60 Rose Carr, "Behind the sciences: AGEs — the everyday substances that age us," HealthyFood, https://www.healthyfood.com/advice/behind-the-science-ages-the-everyday-substances-that-age-us/.

61 Minju Sim et al., "Hydrogen-Rich Water Reduces Inflammatory Responses and Prevents Apoptosis of Peripheral Blood Cells in Healthy Adults: A Randomized, Double-Blind, Controlled Trial," Scientific Reports, July 22, 2020, https://www.nature.com/articles/s41598-020-68930-2?utm_source=convertkit&utm_medium=email&utm_campaign=Optimize%20Your%20Water%20Quality%20and%20Intake%20for%20Health%20-%2010856222.

62 "A good night's sleep is critical for good health," CDC Archive, February 18, 2016, https://archive.cdc.gov/www_cdc_gov/media/releases/2016/p0215-enough-sleep.html.

63 "New study helps explain links between sleep loss and diabetes," February 19, 2015, https://www.uchicagomedicine.org/forefront/news/new-study-helps-explain-links-between-sleep-loss-and-diabetes.

64 "Sleep and the Immune System," March 31, 2020, https://www.cdc.gov/niosh/work-hour-training-for-nurses/longhours/mod2/05.html.

65 Steven Marshall, "Sleep Statistics and Facts," National Council on Aging, March 7, 2024, https://www.ncoa.org/adviser/sleep/sleep-statistics/.

66 Amneet Sandhu, "Daylight savings time and myocardial infarction," Open heart 1, no. 1 (2014), https://pmc.ncbi.nlm.nih.gov/articles/PMC4189320/.

67 Evan MacDonald, "Losing sleep with Daylight Savings Time change could be bad for your health. Here's what will help," Houston Chronicle, March 9, 2023, https://www.houstonchronicle.com/news/houston-texas/health/article/daylight-saving-time-heart-attacks-sleep-17827656.php

68 Danielle Pacheco et al., "Lack of Sleep May Increase Calorie Consumption," Sleep Foundation, December 22, 2023, https://www.sleepfoundation.org/sleep-deprivation/lack-sleep-may-increase-calorie-consumption.

69 Rob Newsom et al., "Slow-Wave Sleep," Sleep Foundation, May 15, 2023, https://www.sleepfoundation.org/stages-of-sleep/slow-wave-sleep.

70 "New Study Finds Deep Sleep Is Best for Brain 'Cleaning,' Shows Connection Between Sleep and Alzheimer's," US Against Alzheimer's, March 1, 2019, https://www.usagainstalzheimers.org/blog/new-study-deep-sleep-best-for-brain-cleaning.

71 S. Groch et al., "The role of REM sleep in the processing of emotional memories: evidence from behavior and event-related potentials," Neurobiology of learning and memory, no. 99 (2013), https://pubmed.ncbi.nlm.nih.gov/23123802/.

72 Jing Zhang et al., "Evidence of an active role of dreaming in emotional memory processing shows that we dream to forget," Sci Rep 14, (2024), https://www.nature.com/articles/s41598-024-58170-z.

73 Christine Blume et al.,"Effects of light on human circadian rhythms, sleep and mood," Somnologie : Schlafforschung und Schlafmedizin = Somnology : sleep research and sleep medicine 23, no. 3 (2019), https://pmc.ncbi.nlm.nih.gov/articles/PMC6751071/.

74 Sharon Brandwein, "Chronotypes: Understanding Types & Impact on Sleep," Sleepopolis, October 26, 2023, https://sleepopolis.com/education/chronotypes/.

75 Jennifer Larson, "What Are Alpha Brain Waves and Why Are They Important?" October 9, 2019, https://www.healthline.com/health/alpha-brain-waves#what-are-they.

76 Giuseppe Barbato, "REM Sleep: An Unknown Indicator of Sleep Quality," International journal of environmental research and public 18, no. 24 (2021), healthhttps://pmc.ncbi.nlm.nih.gov/articles/PMC8702162/.

77 Jan Grzegorzewski, "Pharmacokinetics of Caffeine: A Systematic Analysis of Reported Data for Application in Metabolic Phenotyping and Liver Function Testing," February 24, 2022, https://www.frontiersin.org/journals/pharmacology/articles/10.3389/fphar.2021.752826/full.

78 E. Spindel, "Effects of caffeine on anterior pituitary and thyroid function in the rat," The Journal of pharmacology and experimental therapeutics 214, no. 1 (1980), https://pubmed.ncbi.nlm.nih.gov/6104718/

79 "Neuropsychology: Power naps produce a significant improvement in memory performance," University Saarland, March 20, 2015, https://www.sciencedaily.com/releases/2015/03/150320091315.htm.

80 Joanne Lewsley, "Food coma: What to know about postprandial somnolence," Medical News Today, June 16, 2023, https://www.medicalnewstoday.com/articles/food-coma#causes.

81 Ahmad Afaghi et al.,"Acute effects of the very low carbohydrate diet on sleep indices," Nutritional neuroscience 11, no. 4 (2008), https://pubmed.ncbi.nlm.nih.gov/18681982/.

82 Jill Zwarensteyn, "Inclined Bed Therapy for Sleep Quality: A Detailed Overview," Sleep Advisor, September 10, 2024, https://www.sleepadvisor.org/inclined-bed-therapy/.

83 Joni Sweet, "Why A Sleep Schedule Could Change Your Life," Sleep.com, January 4, 2024, https://www.sleep.com/sleep-health/sleep-schedule.

84 Shannon L. Risacher, PhD et al., "Association Between Anticholinergic

Medication Use and Cognition, Brain Metabolism, and Brain Atrophy in Cognitively Normal Older Adults," JAMA Network, (2016), https://jamanetwork.com/journals/jamaneurology/fullarticle/2514553.

85 "Preschoolers exposed to nighttime light lack melatonin," ScienceDaily, March 5, 2018. https://www.sciencedaily.com/releases/2018/03/180305160151.htm.

86 Annie Price, "Sarcopenia: 10 Keys to Keep Your Muscle Mass Up as You Age," Dr. Axe, October 9, 2024, https://draxe.com/health/sarcopenia/.

87 Humza Siddiqui MD, "Strength Training over 60 Can Help Prevent Sarcopenia," UT Southwestern Medical Center, January 6, 2023, https://utswmed.org/medblog/age-related-sarcopenia/.

88 "The Dangers of Sitting," Better Health Channel, July 2023, https://www.betterhealth.vic.gov.au/health/healthyliving/the-dangers-of-sitting.

89 Agata Blaszczak-Boxe, "Two Hours of Sitting Cancels Out 20 Minutes of Exercise, Study Finds," CBS News, July 8, 2014, https://www.cbsnews.com/news/two-hours-of-sitting-cancels-out-20-minutes-of-exercise-study-finds/.

90 Amira Klip et al., "Thirty Sweet Years of GLUT4," Journal of Biological Chemistry 294, no. 30 (2019), https://www.jbc.org/article/S0021-9258%2820%2930642-6/fulltext.

91 "Exercise Heart Rate Zones Explained," Cleveland Clinic, December 12, 2023. https://health.clevelandclinic.org/exercise-heart-rate-zones-explained/.

92 "Physical Activity," World Health Organization, June 26, 2024, https://www.who.int/news-room/fact-sheets/detail/physical-activity.

93 Ibid.

94 "Anaerobic Exercise," Physiopedia, https://www.physio-pedia.com/Anaerobic_Exercise.

95 Lauretta El Hayek et al., "Lactate Mediates the Effects of Exercise on Learning and Memory through SIRT1-Dependent Activation of Hippocampal Brain-Derived Neurotrophic Factor (BDNF)," The Journal of neuroscience: the official journal of the Society for Neuroscience 39, no. 13 (2019): 2369-2382, https://pmc.ncbi.nlm.nih.gov/articles/PMC6435829/.

96 Matthieu Clauss, "Dietary Polyphenols and Their Impact on Gut

Microbiota in Relation to Human Health," Frontiers in Nutrition 8 (2021), https://www.frontiersin.org/journals/nutrition/articles/10.3389/fnut.2021.637010/full.

97 Vincenzo Monda et al, "Exercise Modifies the Gut Microbiota with Positive Health Effects," Oxidative Medicine and Cellular Longevity 2017, (2017), https://pmc.ncbi.nlm.nih.gov/articles/PMC5357536/#:~:text=Furthermore%20fit%20individuals%20showed%20a,of%20gut%20health%20%5B71%5D.

98 Sun, Chan, Lin, Wu. "Dietary Polyphenols."

99 Alicia Lasek, "High-Intensity Training for Elders: Norwegian Study Gives It a Thumbs Up," McKnight's Long-Term Care News, October 8, 2020, https://www.mcknights.com/news/high-intensity-training-for-elders-norwegian-study-gives-it-a-thumbs-up/.

100 Greg Nuckols, "How many additional calories does each pound of muscle burn?" Stronger by Science, June 14, 2023, https://www.strongerbyscience.com/calories-muscle-burn/.

101 Luc J. C. van Loon, "Role of dietary protein in post-exercise muscle reconditioning," Nestle Nutrition Institute workshop series 75, (2013): 73-83, https://pubmed.ncbi.nlm.nih.gov/23765352/.

102 Sarah Katz. "Fact or Fiction: The Anabolic Window," Lewis College, October 13, 2021. https://lewis.gsu.edu/2021/10/13/fact-or-fiction-the-anabolic-window/.

103 "Falls and Fractures in Older Adults: Causes and Prevention," National Institute on Aging, August 24, 2023, https://www.nia.nih.gov/health/falls-and-falls-prevention/falls-and-fractures-older-adults-causes-and-prevention.

104 Kristin L. Szuhany et al., "A meta-analytic review of the effects of exercise on brain-derived neurotrophic factor," Journal of Psychiatric Research 60, (2015): 56-54, https://pmc.ncbi.nlm.nih.gov/articles/PMC4314337/.

105 Abdallah Mohammad Ibrahim et al., "Brain-Derived Neurotropic Factor in Neurodegenerative Disorders," Biomedicines 10, no. 5 (2022), https://pmc.ncbi.nlm.nih.gov/articles/PMC9138678/.

106 Victor Toro et al., "Effects of Twelve Sessions of High-Temperature Sauna Baths on Body Composition in Healthy Young Men,"

International journal of environmental research and public health 18, no. 9 (2021), https://pmc.ncbi.nlm.nih.gov/articles/PMC8122786/.

107 Rhonda P. Patrick, "Sauna use as a lifestyle practice to extend healthspan," ScienceDirect 154, (2021), https://www.sciencedirect.com/science/article/pii/S0531556521002916.

108 "Practical Guide to Tabata Intervals," Elevate Fitness, https://elevatesyracuse.com/practical-guide-to-tabata-intervals/.

109 "Why Elite Rowers Have Bigger, Stronger Hearts," ScienceDaily, August 15, 2008, https://www.sciencedaily.com/releases/2008/08/080807222006.htm.

110 "The Mind-Body-Spirit Connection," Bruce Lipton: Mind-Body-Spirit Connection, 2023, https://www.brucelipton.com/mind-body-spirit-connection/.

111 Katie Byron, Loving What Is, Revised Edition: Four Questions That Can Change Your Life; The Revolutionary Process Called "The Work" (Harmony, 2021).

112 "The Internal Family Systems Model Outline," IFS Institute, https://ifs-institute.com/resources/articles/internal-family-systems-model-outline.

113 "Why Laughing Is Good for You," Cleveland Clinic, November 11, 2022, https://health.clevelandclinic.org/is-laughing-good-for-you.

114 Hanan Parvez, "How TV Influences Your Mind Through Hypnosis," PsychMechanics, July 13, 2024, https://www.psychmechanics.com/how-tv-influences-your-mind-through/.

115 "The Sound of Music," National Poll on Healthy Aging, February, 2024, https://www.healthyagingpoll.org/reports-more/report/sound-music#xd_co_f=ZmUxOGNlY2YtMjY0MS00M2JmLWFkNmUtZWE0YWIxMjhmOTQz~.

116 Ibid.

117 "Welcome to The Tapping Solution," The Tapping Solution, 2023, https://www.thetappingsolution.com.

118 Dr. Christian Poensgen, "How Panoramic Vision Helps You Destress in Real-Time," Beyond Productivity, January 19, 2023, https://beyondproductivity.substack.com/p/how-panoramic-vision-helps-you-destress.

119 Nikolai A. Shevchuk, "Adapted cold shower as a potential treatment for depression," Medical hypotheses 70, no. 5 (2008): 995-1001m https://pubmed.ncbi.nlm.nih.gov/17993252/.

120 "23 Writing Down Goals Statistics, Facts and Trends in 2024," Dream Maker, July 6, 2024, https://dreammakerr.com/writing-down-goals-statistics/.

121 "Application Form," Your Wellness Made Simple, 2023, https://yourwellness-madesimple.com/application-form/.

To help you maximize your transformation, I have created a library of additional resources just for you.

- Exclusive Recipes
- Quick Guides
- Scientific Sources

Live Well,
Adriana

Scan the QR code below to access everything you need to support your health journey.

LV Book Resources

WELCOME TO YOUR KITCHEN ADVENTURE

Each ingredient in these recipes is chosen with intention to support your vibrant health and well-being. Cooking is a creative process, and I encourage you to use your imagination. Feel free to modify the vegetables, herbs, and spices according to your preferences. Make the kitchen your playground—enjoy the process, and let it be a joyful experience.

To help you get started, here are a few tips that work for me, which I hope will inspire you to build your own routines:

PRODUCE

Visit your local farmers' market for fresh, organic, and local ingredients. To clean produce, fill the sink with cold water, a splash of vinegar, and a teaspoon of baking soda to remove toxins. After rinsing and drying, chop and store for easy access throughout the week. Save scraps like carrot greens or onion skins for making veggie broth.

MEAL PREP ROUTINE

- Make two dressings each week.
- Plan five or more favorite meals to rotate each week.
- Batch cook vegetable soups and hummus, and marinate proteins in advance for easy weekday meals.
- Prep breakfasts such as chia pudding, pancakes, or hard-boiled eggs so you're ready to start your day.

Embrace the joy of cooking and let each step nourish your creativity, bringing vibrant health into your life.

For additional recipes, visit my website at https://yourwellness-madesimple.com

SWEET AND CRISPY GRANOLA

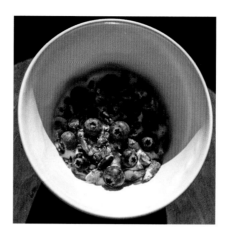

INGREDIENTS

½ cup unsweetened
  coconut flakes
½ cup chopped walnuts
½ cup chopped pecans
2 tablespoons
  pumpkin seeds
2 tablespoons chia seeds
6 Brazil nuts, chopped
¼ cup cocoa nibs
1 teaspoon ghee,
  room temperature
1 teaspoon ground cinnamon

1 teaspoon vanilla extract
1 teaspoon high-quality
  pure salt

1 teaspoon ground ginger
(optional)
1 teaspoon ground cloves
(optional)
1 teaspoon ground
cardamom (optional)
½ cup bee pollen (optional)
1 tablespoon honey (optional)

DIRECTIONS

1. Preheat the oven to 250 degrees.

2. Mix the coconut flakes, walnuts, pecans, pumpkin seeds, chia seeds, Brazil nuts, salt, cinnamon, vanilla extract, and cocoa nibs together.
3. Stir optional spices into ghee, if using. Add ghee to nut mixture and mix well.
4. Line a baking sheet with parchment paper and spread the mixture evenly on the pan.
5. Bake 15 minutes. Take out, stir, and then bake for another 15 minutes.
6. Allow the granola to cool completely. Mix in the bee pollen and honey, if desired.
7. Serve with yogurt or kefir and berries. Store any leftovers in a glass airtight container in the fridge.

Note: I recommend purchasing already sprouted, organic nuts and seeds.

BRIGHT AND FILLING YOGURT BOWL

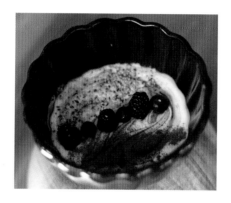

INGREDIENTS

1 (0.5-ounce) scoop whey
protein powder

1 (0.4-ounce) scoop
collagen powder

1 cup grass-fed plain yogurt
or sheepmilk yogurt

1 tablespoon pistachio butter
or hazelnut butter

1 tablespoon hemp hearts

½ cup fresh blueberries

1 teaspoon cinnamon

DIRECTIONS

1. Put one scoop of protein powder and collagen powder into a bowl with the yogurt.
2. Stir until well combined.
3. Add the nut butter and cinnamon and gently swirl them in.
4. Top with hemp hearts and blueberries and enjoy.

APPLE PANCAKE WITH WHIPPED CREAM AND HONEY

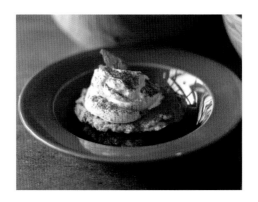

INGREDIENTS

2 red apples

1 teaspoon vanilla extract

1 teaspoon baking powder

2 eggs

½ cup almond flour

Extra Virgin Olive Oil
(for frying)

Whipped cream (for topping)

1 teaspoon honey (for
drizzling)

Nut butter (optional, for extra
richness)

Berries (optional, for
freshness)

1 (0.5-ounce) scoop of
collagen or whey protein
powder (optional, for more
protein)

DIRECTIONS

1. Shred the red apples and squeeze out all excess liquid
   using a clean kitchen towel or cheesecloth.

2. In a medium bowl combine the shredded apples with the vanilla extract, baking powder, eggs, almond flour, and optional scoop of collagen powder. Mix everything well with a fork until the batter is evenly combined.
3. Heat a skillet over medium heat and add a small amount of Extra Virgin Olive Oil.
4. Spoon the batter into the pan to form pancakes of your desired size.
5. Cook each pancake for about 2 to 3 minutes on each side.
6. Top each pancake with a spoonful of whipped cream.
7. Drizzle with honey. Add a dollop of nut butter or a handful of fresh berries for extra flavor and texture.

CREAMY SALMON WITH HUMMUS

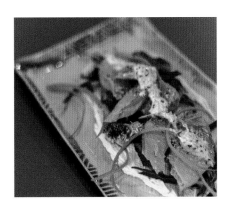

INGREDIENTS

1 cup white bean hummus
  (see recipe below)

1 cup shredded red cabbage

1 cup thinly shredded carrots

1 cup cooked broccoli florets

1 6-ounce cooked
  salmon fillet

Juice of ½ a lemon

1 tablespoon Extra Virgin
  Olive Oil

¼ cup tzatziki sauce

2 tablespoons hemp seeds

½ cup of cold water

WHITE BEAN HUMMUS

INGREDIENTS

1 (15-ounce) can white beans,
  drained and rinsed

½ cup cauliflower florets

1 teaspoon baking soda

½ teaspoon ground cumin

Juice of 1 lemon

1 garlic clove, peeled
  and in half

2 tablespoons tahini

¼ cup Extra Virgin Olive Oil

2 teaspoons salt

½ cup of cold water

DIRECTIONS

For the hummus

1. In a medium saucepan combine the drained white beans, cauliflower florets, garlic, and baking soda.
2. Cover with water and bring to a boil. Reduce the heat and simmer for about 10 minutes, until the cauliflower is tender.
3. Strain the beans, cauliflower, and garlic, then transfer them to a high-speed blender or food processor.
4. Add the lemon juice, tahini, salt, cumin, and olive oil.
5. Blend until smooth, adding cold water gradually to achieve your desired consistency.
6. Taste the hummus and adjust the lemon juice, salt, or spices as needed for flavor.

For the salmon

1. Spread 3 to 5 tablespoons of hummus on a serving plate.
2. On top of the hummus, layer the shredded cabbage, shredded carrots, and cooked broccoli.
3. Place the cooked salmon on top of the vegetables.
4. Squeeze the fresh lemon juice over the entire plate.
5. Drizzle with the Extra Virgin Olive Oil to add richness and flavor.
6. Drizzle with the tzatziki sauce.
7. Sprinkle with hemp seeds for added texture and nutrition, and serve.

PAPRIKA CHICKEN

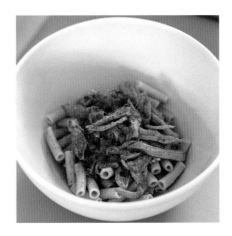

INGREDIENTS

1 tablespoon olive oil

3 medium onions, chopped

2 tablespoons paprika

5 pounds chicken thighs,
bone-in, skinless

Water, to cover

Salt, to taste

Cooked pasta or rice

Chopped garlic chives
for garnish

DIRECTIONS

1. In a large pot add the oil, chopped onions, and a pinch of salt.
2. Cover the pot and cook the onions on medium-low heat for 15 to 20 minutes, stirring occasionally, until they become soft and release their juices.
3. Once the onions are softened and juicy, stir in the paprika. Mix well to ensure the onions are evenly coated.

4. Place the chicken thighs into the pot with the onion mixture.
5. Stir to coat the chicken with the onions and paprika.
6. Add water just to cover the chicken. Cover the pot and cook on medium-low heat for about 45 minutes until the chicken is fully cooked and tender.
7. Remove the chicken thighs from the pot and let them cool slightly.
8. Pick the meat off the bones, shred it, and return the shredded chicken to the pot. Mix it well with the onion sauce.
9. Serve the paprika chicken over your choice of pasta or rice with chopped garlic chives.

MEDITERRANEAN WILD MEATBALLS WITH TZATZIKI

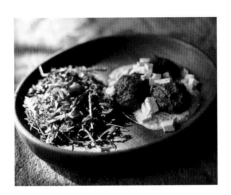

INGREDIENTS

For the meatballs

1 pound ground bison

1 pound ground lamb

2 eggs

2 tablespoons ground flaxseed

1 tablespoon onion powder

1 tablespoon fresh oregano, chopped

1 tablespoon dried sage

1 teaspoon dried marjoram

1 tablespoon chopped fresh rosemary

1 tablespoon salt

3 garlic cloves, minced

½ cup crumbled feta cheese

For the salad

1 large handful lettuce leaves

2 cups shredded vegetables (whatever you prefer)

Juice of 1 lemon

1 tablespoon apple cider vinegar

2 tablespoons Extra Virgin Olive Oil

Salt, to taste

DIRECTIONS

1. Preheat your oven to 325 degrees and line a baking sheet with parchment paper.
2. In a large mixing bowl combine the bison, lamb, eggs, flaxseed, spices, and garlic.
3. Form the mixture into meatballs, about 2 inches in diameter, and place them on the prepared baking sheet.
4. Bake for 20 to 25 minutes, or until the meatballs are cooked through.
5. While the meatballs are baking, prepare the tzatziki sauce and refrigerate.
6. In a large salad bowl combine your shredded vegetables with the lemon juice, apple cider vinegar, olive oil, and salt. Toss to coat the vegetables evenly. Lightly mix in the lettuce leaves.
7. Serve the meatballs over a spoonful of yogurt tzatziki sauce. Garnish with crumbled feta cheese.
8. Serve the salad on the side.

SPROUT SALAD WITH THRIVE DRESSING

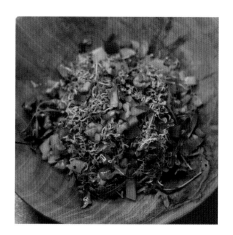

INGREDIENTS

For the dressing

1-inch piece fresh
  ginger, peeled

1 small shallot, peeled

1 teaspoon whole cori-
  ander seeds

1 teaspoon whole
  cumin seeds

Juice of 1 lemon

2 tablespoons apple cider
  vinegar

2 tablespoons balsamic
  vinegar

½ cup olive oil

Salt, to taste

For the salad

½ yellow bell pepper, diced

½ red bell pepper, diced

1 cup arugula leaves

1 cup mixed sprouts (such as
  alfalfa, broccoli, or radish
  sprouts)

3 tablespoons thinly sliced
  green onions

1 handful crushed walnuts
  or pecans

DIRECTIONS

For the dressing

1. Place all the dressing ingredients in a high-speed blender and blend until smooth.
2. Adjust the taste as you wish with salt and acidity.

For the salad

1. Gently toss all the ingredients together until well combined. Dress with the dressing.
2. Serve immediately as a fresh and healthy side dish or light meal.

MUSHROOM FRIED RICE

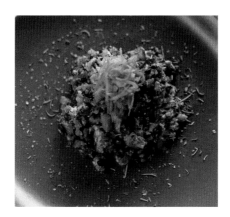

INGREDIENTS

1 large onion, chopped

3 garlic cloves

3 medium carrots, chopped

2 cups mushrooms, finely chopped

2 teaspoons grated fresh ginger

1 teaspoon ground cumin

1 teaspoon ground turmeric

1 cup dry California wild rice

2 eggs

2 green onions, sliced

½ cup broccoli sprouts

2 tablespoons kimchi

2 tablespoons shredded manchego cheese (optional)

DIRECTIONS

1. Rinse the rice and soak it for 2 hours or overnight. Cook the rice according to the package instructions. (Optional: After the rice is cooked, cool it down in the fridge overnight, if possible, to create resistant starch.

2. In a stainless steel skillet or wok, sauté the onions, garlic, carrots, and mushrooms until soft.
3. Stir in the grated ginger, cumin, and turmeric and cook for a few minutes.
4. Add the cooked rice and stir well.
5. Make a well in the middle, exposing the hot pan, and add the eggs. Scramble the eggs with a spatula until cooked, then fold the rice through to incorporate. Stir everything together for a few more seconds and remove from the heat.
6. Garnish with the green onions, sprouts, and kimchi, and serve with shredded Manchego cheese on top if you wish.

CREAMY LEMON BELL PEPPERS

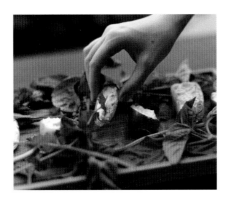

INGREDIENTS

12 mini bell peppers

3 ounces soft goat cheese

8 ounces ricotta cheese

Zest of 1 lemon

Juice of 1 lemon

1 garlic clove, pressed

1 handful fresh basil
    leaves, chopped

1 shallot, finely chopped

1 teaspoon Italian seasoning

1 teaspoon dried dill

Salt, to taste

DIRECTIONS

1. Wash the mini bell peppers and carefully remove the seeds and membranes from the insides.
2. In a medium-sized mixing bowl, combine the goat cheese and ricotta cheese.
3. Add the lemon zest lemon juice garlic, basil, shallot, Italian seasoning, dill, and salt.
4. Carefully fill each mini bell pepper with the cheese mixture and enjoy with a fresh arugula salad or your favorite salad.

IRRESISTIBLE MASH WITH MUSHROOMS

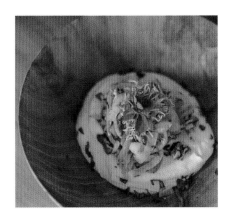

INGREDIENTS

1 medium cauliflower, chopped

1 celery root, cubed

½ package soft goat cheese (or 1 tablespoon apple cider vinegar if not using cheese)

Salt, to taste

1 large onion, thinly sliced

1 cup shitake mushrooms (or your favorite), sliced

Juice of ½ a lemon

1 handful broccoli sprouts

Dried herbs of choice, for sprinkling

Extra virgin olive oil, for drizzling

Balsamic vinegar, for drizzling

Sliced avocado (optional)

Sunny-side up egg (optional)

DIRECTIONS

1. Steam the cauliflower and cubed celery root until tender, about 10 minutes.

2. Heat a large skillet over medium heat and add the onion with a little water and salt. Cover and cook until soft but not browned (approximately 20 minutes). Stir occasionally to avoid caramelization.
3. In a blender or with a hand mixer, blend the cauliflower and celery root together with the cheese (or apple cider vinegar if not using cheese) and salt until smooth.
4. Once the onions are softened, add the mushrooms to the skillet. Cook until the mushrooms are tender, about 5 to 10 minutes.
5. Once the onions and mushrooms are done, drizzle with lemon juice.
6. Plate the cauliflower and celery root mash, top with the sautéed onions and mushrooms, and sprinkle with the broccoli sprouts and dried herbs. Drizzle with theextra virgin olive oil.
7. Optionally, add sliced avocado or a sunny-side up egg.
8. Finish with a drizzle of balsamic vinegar and serve immediately.

TZATZIKI SAUCE

INGREDIENTS

1 cup sheep milk yogurt or
   Greek yogurt

1 cucumber, grated and
   squeezed to remove water

1 tablespoon fresh
   lemon juice

1 tablespoon chopped
   fresh dill

1 garlic clove, minced

Salt, to taste

DIRECTIONS

In a medium bowl, stir all the ingredients together until well
blended. Refrigerate if not using immediately.

DRESSINGS

For nearly all these dressings, the directions are the same: Combine all the ingredients in a blender or food processor and blend until smooth. Store in an airtight container in the fridge and shake well before using. Enjoy!

BASIL-GINGER DRESSING

INGREDIENTS

½ cup apple cider vinegar

½ cup water

1-inch piece of fresh ginger, peeled and chopped

1 shallot, chopped

½ garlic clove, minced

Juice of 1 lemon

1 handful fresh basil leaves

Salt, to taste

DIRECTIONS

Blend well in a blender and enjoy!

MINT-DILL DRESSING

INGREDIENTS

½ cup apple cider vinegar

½ cup water

1 shallot, chopped

½ garlic clove, minced

Juice of 1 lemon

1 handful fresh mint leaves

1 handful fresh dill

Salt, to taste

DIRECTIONS

Blend well in a blender and enjoy!

CILANTRO-LIME DRESSING

INGREDIENTS

½ cup apple cider vinegar

½ cup water

1 shallot, chopped

½ garlic clove, minced

Juice of 1 lime

1 handful fresh cilantro leaves

Salt, to taste

DIRECTIONS

Blend well in a blender and enjoy!

TAHINI HERB DRESSING

INGREDIENTS

3 tablespoons tahini

2 tablespoons apple cider vinegar

1 shallot, finely chopped

½ teaspoon paprika

½ teaspoon dried rosemary, crushed

¼ cup olive oil

Salt, to taste

Water, as needed (to adjust consistency)

DIRECTIONS

Blend well in a blender and enjoy!

CREAMY FETA DRESSING

INGREDIENTS

1 (8-ounce) container
   feta cheese
2 tablespoons extra virgin
   olive oil
Juice of ½ a lemon

1 small garlic clove, minced
2 teaspoons dried oregano
1 handful cauliflower
   florets, steamed

DIRECTIONS

Blend the mixture until it becomes smooth and creamy.

COTTAGE CHEESE HERB DRESSING

INGREDIENTS

2 cups cottage cheese
1 handful artichoke hearts
   (squeeze the water out if
   using canned)
1 teaspoon dried cilantro

1 teaspoon dried dill
1 teaspoon garlic powder
½ teaspoon onion powder
¼ teaspoon salt
Juice of ½ a lemon

DIRECTIONS

Blend well in a blender and enjoy!

GUMMIES

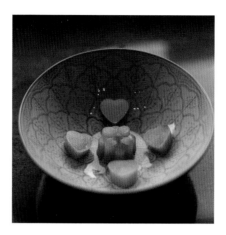

INGREDIENTS

4 tablespoons gelatin   1 cup water

1 cup fruit or vegetable juice   1 cup berries, pureed

2 tablespoons lemon juice

DIRECTIONS

1. Pour the gelatin into the bottom of a medium-sized saucepan.
2. Pour the pureed berries, fruit or vegetable juice, lemon juice, and water over the gelatin and, using a fork, mix well. It will make a thick paste—just keep mixing until there are no lumps.
3. Heat the mixture over a low flame until the mixture melts and becomes clear.
4. Pour the mixture into a gummy bear mold or other silicone mold. It will be easier if you transfer from the

    saucepan to a small pitcher or measuring cup with a pour spout.

5. To speed up the cooling and hardening process, you can put your molds in the refrigerator until cool.

6. Once the gummy shapes have cooled and hardened, pop them out of the molds. They will keep in a jar or other container in the refrigerator for about a week (if they last that long!).

Note: Adding the gelatin too quickly will make it more diffi-cult to get the mixture to incorporate. An immersion blender is not necessary but greatly speeds up the process.

SMOOTH CHOCOLATE MOUSSE

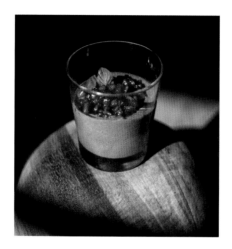

INGREDIENTS

2 tablespoons chia seeds

1 (0.5-ounce) scoop
   whey protein

1 (0.2-ounce) scoop cocoa
   powder (or CocoaVia)

½ cup nut or goat milk

1 teaspoon vanilla extract

1 teaspoon honey

Pomegranate seeds and
   blueberries to top

Plain yogurt to top (optional)

DIRECTIONS

1. Blend chia seeds, whey protein, cocoa powder, milk, vanilla, and honey well in a high-speed blender.
2. Let the mousse sit for three hours or overnight refrigerated in a glass jar.
3. Top with fruit and yogurt, if desired, and serve.

SHREDDED CHICKEN RICE SOUP

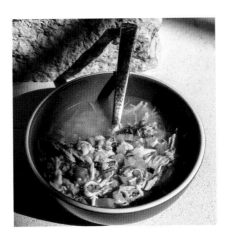

INGREDIENTS

1 tablespoon olive oil

3 medium carrots, peeled
 and sliced

1 leek, chopped

3 celery ribs, sliced

1 onion, diced

4 garlic cloves, minced

1 tablespoon salt

1 tablespoon dried thyme

1 tablespoon dried tarragon

1 tablespoon dried rosemary

1 tablespoon dried oregano

1 cup California wild rice (or
 sorghum or buckwheat if
 desired)

2 boneless skinless chicken
 breasts

5 cups broth or water

Broccoli sprouts, optional

DIRECTIONS

1. In a large soup pot, heat the olive oil over medium heat
   and sauté the carrots, leek, celery, and onion for 10
   minutes.

2. Add the garlic, salt, and herbs, and mix well.
3. Add the rice and mix well.
4. Add the chicken and water. Bring to a boil, then reduce the heat to low and cover the pot. Simmer the soup for thirty minutes, or until the chicken is fully cooked.
5. With tongs, remove the chicken to a cutting board and gently shred the chicken with two forks or a standing mixer. Place the shredded chicken back into the pot and simmer for an additional 1 to 2 minutes.
6. Top with broccoli sprouts and enjoy.

THE ONE:
DODKO'S SOUP

I share this soup in memory of a dear friend, Joseph (Dodko), who passed during the writing of this book. If I could see him again, I'd tell him: *I miss you. I knew I couldn't give you a healthy, longer life. All I wanted was to ease your pain.*

I felt a calling. It wasn't a thought; it was an instinct. I was sitting at the dining room table in California with my family, having lunch. Many years back, we went to Slovakia for Christmas. The flight back was scary due to snow and wind. I vowed never to fly to Slovakia in the winter again. But here you were, calling me to come.

It was the fall of 2023. "We are going to Slovakia for Christmas!" I announced. It just came out of me. My daughter's eyes lit up, and she had a huge smile. "*Yes!*" My husband frowned, though it's not unusual for him not to be excited about new ideas.

We are going to Slovakia. It's clear!

I was going for two reasons: to be with my best friend Joseph (Dodko) who was calling me energetically, and to finally cut the cord from my mother. I had been working through trauma on my own in California and was ready to close a big chapter with her. We must heal the wounds placed on our shoulders and in our hearts as children so we can live freely and truly.

Dodko and I were opposites in many ways, yet so close. Early in his diagnosis, he didn't want to give up his lifestyle; he wanted a miracle pill to continue with his lifestyle as usual. He trusted the doctors. When he was ready to change in

December 2023, with metastasis in his brain, it was too late. I did all he asked, but it was too late.

The traumas we carry, our food and drink habits, our sleep and exercise patterns all have consequences. With respect, we all have our journeys in life, as my dear friend had. I had to respect his journey and be there for him until the end.

In honor of the one who was so hard to open up, who challenged me to dig deep until he did open up, who always had a smile on his face, collected elephants for good luck, loved all animals and nature, and loved his family deeply.

The one who stayed up late, loved music more than anyone I know, loved to drink beer and hruskovica (pear hard liquor) too much, loved mushroom foraging, loved to cook for people with rich flavors, and loved pork knuckle (bravcove koleno) more than any other food.

The one who knew me, the one who loved me. My true soul friend. We had so much fun together, so many deep, great conversations over more than twenty years.

I was blessed with this gift—to have a friend with such deep love, respect, and appreciation. It was this true relationship that made my world a better place to live in.

He was there for my lowest and highest moments, including when I decided to leave my country. He and my other close friends helped me escape. He was there through all the joys and pains.

Dear Dodko, you had a smile that could light up the room. You savored life's simple pleasures. But above all, you knew me and loved me for my truest self. Our connection was deep and unbreakable, a bond that transcended words and filled my heart with gratitude. As I say goodbye, I carry the memories of our time together.

Thank you, my dear friend, for blessing my life with your presence.

I'll remember you holding my hand and kissing me with tears in your eyes on the ride to oncology in December 2023. I'll always remember holding you tight. I am so blessed to have been loved by you and to have loved someone like you.

Thank you for coming to my dreams before you left. Thank you for talking to me throughout the last few weeks before you left this Earth. I knew you carried a lot of regret, pain, and sorrow. I know, Dodko, you are free now. I feel your free energy.

This dish is for you.

It was Wednesday night in California, Thursday at 2:30 a..m. in Slovakia, when you left this earth. I had one more day of photoshoot of my recipes for this book. I finished as planned on Thursday night. Early Friday morning, still dark, you pulled me into the kitchen to make one more dish, for you. Here it is, The One. This is in honor of you and for you, and I know many will enjoy it!

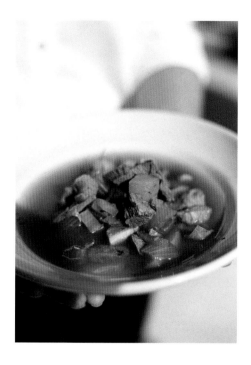

INGREDIENTS

1 large onion

4 garlic cloves

2 stalks celery

1 celery root

2 carrots

16 ounces bison steak

1 tablespoon dried rosemary

1 tablespoon dried sage

1 tablespoon dried thyme

1 tablespoon salt, adjusted
    to taste

6 cups water—enough to
    cover all the ingredients

DIRECTIONS

1. Chop vegetables in chunky pieces, around a half inch big.
2. Place all ingredients in the pot of a slow cooker and cook on low for 2 hours.